*This book is dedicated to my wife, Noureen,
and my amazing daughters, Miraal and Misha.
Family is everything to me,
and I hope you are as proud of me as I am of you!*

CONTENTS

UPGRADE YOUR YOUR VAGUS NERVE

CONTROL INFLAMMATION,
BOOST IMMUNE RESPONSE,
AND IMPROVE HEART RATE VARIABILITY
WITH NEW SCIENCE-BACKED THERAPIES

DR. NAVAZ HABIB

Published by:
Ulysses Press
PO Box 3440
Berkeley, CA 94703
www.ulyssespress.com

ISBN: 978-1-64604-618-8
Library of Congress Control Number: 2023943924

Printed in the United States
10 9 8 7 6 5 4 3 2 1

Project editor: Renee Rutledge
Managing editor: Claire Chun
Editor: Scott Calamar
Front cover design: Rebecca Lown
Interior illustrations: © Tania Sultana except for page 118 phase I and II toxins
    © Ankita; chapter graphics © ya_blue_ko/shutterstock.com
Layout: Winnie Liu

INTRODUCTION

I recently traveled to Los Angeles for my cousin's wedding and stayed with some of my family in a rental home property just north of the city. It was a large home that we were able to lounge in as we took some time away from the chaos of the wedding festivities. There were three bathrooms in the house, and I had a choice of which shower I wanted to use. The shower I chose was the prompt I needed for writing the introduction to this book.

The shower that I used was very difficult to control. It had two knobs, one for hot water and one for cold water. I wasn't particularly in the mood for a cold shower as it was unseasonably cold in California while I was visiting. There was very low water pressure from the shower head, and the temperature control was very sensitive. The slightest excess rotation of either knob resulted in a significant change to the temperature of the water. It was either scalding hot or extremely cold. It also didn't help that if anyone else in the house needed to use the water, the temperature would immediately shift, which made me anxious of all potential scenarios that could result in the water temperature changing drastically.

In the years since I wrote and published my first book, *Activate Your Vagus Nerve*, I have been learning so much more about the exciting research into the effects of the vagus nerve, even more than I thought I knew five years ago! I believe that the more we learn, the more we realize how little we truly know.

All of this amazing new information was the reason I decided to follow up the first book, because I felt that I needed to get more info out to the world as to the importance of an optimally functioning vagus nerve, particularly when it comes to cellular and immune health. The immune system is so much more than the protection system of the body. This is the generic and conventional view of immune system function, one that I feel the need to debunk in this book.

Contrary to popular belief, we as humans actually can control the function of our immune system using our nervous systems, and the vagus nerve is the direct pathway.

The name of the vagus nerve is one of mystery and uncertainty. It literally comes from the root word "vague," in the context of wandering throughout the body, but I also believe that when it was first named, the function of this nerve was mystifying to everyone involved. This nerve was so different from all the other nerves in the body.

Spinal nerves extend from the spinal cord and branch out to innervate skeletal muscles. These nerves signal proprioception (the position of parts of our bodies in space) and movement to and from the brain. They are very important but relatively easy to understand in terms of function.

Sympathetic nerves, an important component of the autonomic nervous system (the neural pathways that control the automatic subconscious functions of our body), extend from the sympathetic chain, a connection of neurons emerging from the brain stem. The sympathetic chain resides on the front sides of the spinal column and have a single nerve branch from the chain to each visceral organ, signaling the fight-or-flight response to stress. We will explore the importance of this system later in this book but know that each of these nerves has a simple and singular connection.

Cranial nerves have functions within the cranial cavity, and as such, generally remain within the head and face region. They are important for many of our senses (sight, smell, hearing, and taste) as well as movement of skeletal muscles in the head and neck. They also send sympathetic and parasympathetic information to and from the cranial region. Without these 12 pairs of nerves extending from the brain stem, we would lack any facial senses or movements.

As the only cranial nerves in the body to extend from the brain stem and into the rest of the body, the vagus nerves have incredibly broad and varying connections throughout the body, send parasympathetic information to and from the visceral organs, and have a very important connection to the sympathetic chain (resulting in control over immune system cells). Yes, I wrote "the vagus *nerves*." Although we commonly refer to it (as I subsequently will) as *the* vagus nerve, we actually have two of them, one on each side of the body. The vagus nerves are unique in that they make up the physical connection of the parasympathetic component of the autonomic nervous system, to and from nearly every single organ in our body.

The vagus nerve is the only nerve in the body with such varying anatomy, connectivity, and important functionality, and I was immediately drawn to it. I've been intrigued by this particular nerve for almost 30 years, ever since I saw the vagus nerve and the connections it had in an anatomy textbook when I was in grade school. The explanation that this nerve, entirely unique from all other nerves in the body, simply was the connection of the parasympathetic nervous system was insufficient to me.

The vast majority of health practitioners don't truly realize the importance of this nerve. We as healthcare providers are given this explanation of parasympathetic control within the body, and then we proceed to overlook the nerve for the rest of our careers. This just isn't good enough for me; thus, I have made it my life's purpose to share this valuable information with the world so that doctors and healthcare practitioners worldwide can provide better care to their patients and clients.

It is my purpose in life to empower healthcare practitioners and health seekers alike to understand that the vagus nerve is the common thread and the physical connection of regulation of homeostasis within the body, and when this nerve is dysfunctional, the result is chronic disease and diagnoses with no known cures. The exciting news is that science and technology are catching up and providing more answers each day as to how vagus nerve function can be measured, improved, and optimized.

Now let's get back to why the idea for the introduction of the book came to me in the shower in Los Angeles.

While fiddling with the knobs to try to find the perfect temperature, I realized that the control of the water being dispensed was dysfunctional and very tricky to get to work correctly. It was extremely hot or extremely cold. It was weaker than I would have liked. It created a minor but palpable psychological and physiological shift in my body.

The shower was dysregulated—dysregulated in the same way that our autonomic nervous system becomes dysregulated. In the same way that the water pressure was low, the tone or signaling power of the vagus nerve can decrease when there is too much pressure or overuse. In the same way that the temperature shifted so easily from hot to cold, parasympathetic and sympathetic control need to be in balance. Without balance, our autonomic state can shift too easily from hot to cold or from fight/flight to rest/digest. My personal fiddling with the temperature knobs created a back-and-forth between hot and cold, but so did external factors that I was not fully aware of or had any ability to control.

The experience I had while taking that shower provided a simple context for me to be able to explain the effect of a dysregulated autonomic nervous system on my ability to take a simple shower.

What our bodies need is effective resilience to change. Homeostasis is not a static state of being, it is a constant ebb and flow between hot and cold, but one that is so effectively fine-tuned, it allows us to only feel warm. The regulation of the autonomic nervous system lies more in the function and effective signaling of the vagus nerve and the parasympathetic nervous system. Our goal should be to increase our adaptive capacity, a concept we will discuss in depth throughout this book.

Imagine that in the shower, the hot water gets turned up or down by the stressors we have experienced, both in the past and day-to-day life. For some people that knob is turned up to the maximum level. Our ability to regulate to a warm temperature is to turn the cold knob up or down actively and consciously until we find a balanced temperature. The quicker and more effective we are at doing this, the less temperature shift we will feel. In our body, the sympathetic nervous system is on high alert (the hot knob is always on), and our ability to keep the temperature warm and comfortable is entirely dependent on the vagus nerve and parasympathetic control.

A dysfunctional vagus nerve results in an overactive and under-controlled stress activation system. The result is excessive inflammation, immune cell activation, cellular dysfunction, and breakdown of the optimal function of our bodies. All chronic life-style diseases that we know about are a result of poor inflammatory control due to a weak or dysfunctional vagus nerve.

In order to support your journey to understand and optimize the function of your vagus nerve, I have created a free workbook that you can use to assess the challenges that are causing vagus nerve dysfunction in your life, to begin measuring the function of the nerve, and to simply and effectively begin adding exercises, tools, and strategies to improve the function of your vagus nerve. You can download this workbook for free at www.vagusnervebook.com.

In Section 1 of this book, we will dig into the stressors and factors that drive sympathetic activation. In this section you can work along with me and identify the specific stressors that have been affecting you and the timeline of events responsible for taking you down this path. In my practice, it has become evident to me that there is a near 100 percent correlation to the symptoms of a chronic condition becoming clear following a particularly stress-ful or challenging event in one's life. Working through the stressor timeline can help you to open your eyes to the specific stressors and understand the cumulative effects of stressors in your life, as well as the potential inciting incident that triggered the symptoms you may be experiencing.

Section 2 will review and discuss the best ways to measure vagus nerve function, including a deeper dive into heart rate variabil-ity and the use of wearable health-monitoring devices. Once we understand the history of how you got to where you are, we can begin taking account of where you currently stand and determine your baseline health markers. We will use this baseline data to help determine steps to move forward and improve our health markers using the techniques discussed in Section 3.

Section 3 will go over specific strategies and tools for improving and optimizing vagus nerve function. We will briefly review foundational exercises that were discussed in my first book, but the focus of this section will be primarily on new research, tools, and devices that show significant promise in creating amazing changes in those suffering from chronic health conditions, and even some that have been shown to improve cognitive function and hack our ability to function for the better!

Do or do not, there is no try. —Master Yoda

I'm honored to share my work and demystify the power of this nerve for you. Throughout this book, I hope to empower you to utilize the best tools available to make the changes necessary to extend your health span and provide you and your family the best that life has to offer!

IDENTIFYING STRESSORS— DOWNGRADING VAGUS NERVE FUNCTION

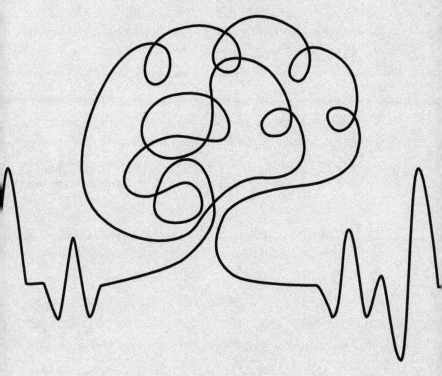

CHAPTER 1

UNDERSTANDING STRESSORS

Let's imagine that your body is like a car, with two pedals—an accelerator and a brake pedal. Most of the time that car is parked with the brakes engaged, so that the car cannot move without someone pushing the accelerator. When you do begin to drive the car, you initially push the brake pedal while shifting into the drive or reverse gears, then push the accelerator to get the car to move in the direction of your choice.

While driving, there will be instances in which higher speeds are necessary, so you push the accelerator a little harder, allowing the car to move at a faster speed—needing to overtake the car beside you, entering a freeway, or simply beginning to move when the traffic light turns green.

There will also be instances in which you need to push the brake—coming to a red light or stop sign, if someone cuts you off, or if you are sitting in bumper-to-bumper traffic during rush hour.

Both pedals are necessary to make the car function well. We need the accelerator when we have to move and make headway to get closer to our goals or complete our tasks, and we need the brakes when we have to stop, giving us control and ensuring that we keep all occupants and pedestrians safe.

This is, in my opinion, a perfect analogy to understand the autonomic nervous system of the human body. Without an accelerator—the sympathetic branch of the autonomic nervous system—we would be unable to move efficiently and effectively through life. Without a brake pedal—the parasympathetic branch of the autonomic nervous system—we would be unable to slow down, control our movements, and stop when necessary.

When both systems are working perfectly—the accelerator sending signals to the engine/motor to move the car at various speeds, and brakes being able to slow us down or stop us efficiently and effectively—we can drive on the road and keep all occupants safe. The steering wheel directs where we want to go in a conscious fashion, so the entire system works in harmony to help us reach our desired destination safely and efficiently.

We must also consider what can happen when the system is not working perfectly, as this is how we head down the path of dysfunction and eventually disease. The key here is *control.* We need to be able to slow down and even stop when necessary, and we need to be able to speed up when that is necessary.

We must too be capable of slowing down and stopping when we feel the need. If a car is going too fast in a school zone, we need to slow down to a safer speed. If another car pulls in front of us in a parking lot, we need to be able to stop so that we don't get into an accident. The brakes of the system impart control to the driver to ensure safety. In the same way, we have a parasympathetic nervous system that slows us down and allows us to be in control of our movements. In order to ensure that this control system is working well, we must have strong brake pads and rotors, as well as brake fluid, so we can send the signals to the wheels that we require to slow down.

Stressors are the factors that help us to push the accelerator and activate the sympathetic nervous system. Traditionally, we have called this the fight-or-flight system, but I believe that this is an incomplete statement. In order to be productive and move toward a goal, we need to activate this system. The sympathetic nervous system is what mobilizes and excites us toward a state of accomplishment. It is the system that pushes us to get up and get going. Just as a car without a functional accelerator cannot move forward toward a destination, a person without a functional sympathetic nervous system would be unable to move toward a goal.

Stress can be both positive and negative. There are two prefixes that change the way we define this word. "Eu-" is the prefix that puts a positive spin on the word, while "di-" creates a negative connotation. Let's consider the definition of the words "eustress" and "distress."

Eustress is any challenge that turns on the sympathetic nervous system and mobilizes you to move toward a personal or professional goal. Training for a marathon or 100-mile bike ride would be considered eustress. Taking on a new client in your business is a positive stressor as it helps push your business toward a revenue or growth goal. When you view an upcoming challenge in a positive light—as a step toward achieving a bigger goal—this is considered eustress. More often than not, eustress is a positive challenge created by ourselves, in our own mind. We set the goal, we create the steps involved, and the universe conspires to put us in a position to overcome these challenges, moving us closer to these goals.

I consider distress to be any challenge that pushes you away or holds you back from achieving a goal. Distress can be created both intrinsically by us but often has an extrinsic source. We then experience this distress internally, affecting our biology and biochemistry in a way that holds us back from moving in a desired direction. Stress is not intrinsically negative, but if we view it through a lens of a challenge that is holding us back from achieving, then it can create a negative cascade and internal strife.

This is particularly true of major acute traumatic incidents and chronic stress, which are life challenges that affect us negatively over a longer period of time.

When stress is traumatic or chronic, it feels like we are pushing both the accelerator and brake pedals at the same time. In doing so, we create a physiological challenge against our ability to control. The accelerator is being pushed so hard that the brake pads begin to wear out. If this happens consistently over a longer period of time, the brakes will wear out completely and the brake system of the car will become significantly less efficient and potentially stop working. In the same way, if the sympathetic nervous system is constantly being turned on due to various sources of chronic distress, the parasympathetic nervous system—primarily the vagus nerve—will burn out and become less effective at imparting control over the mobilized system.

Luckily, we are capable of restoring and rebuilding this system, but it requires some real work to do so.

Step 1 is to identify the sources of stress and classify them into positive and negative stressors.

Step 2 is to understand the vagus nerve, the cholinergic anti-inflammatory pathway, and the parasympathetic nervous system to see just how effective the rest, digest, recover system is truly functioning.

Step 3 is to implement strategies for rebuilding the parasympathetic nervous system that are science backed and highly effective.

First, let's spend some time identifying and classifying stressors that can help us move forward toward a goal (eustress) and those that are commonly holding people back (distress).

CHAPTER 2

DAILY STRESSORS

Let's begin with the type of stressor that we generally refer to as "stress." These are the day-to-day challenges that each of us experiences in varying degrees. Daily stressors can include financial challenges, relational challenges, and work- or business-related challenges.

Whether it's ensuring there is enough cash in your bank account or keeping an eye on your investment portfolio, financial challenges affect most people. This book features zero strategies on eliminating or managing financial stress, but here are a few of my favorite books on this exact topic:

◆ *I Will Teach You to Be Rich* by Ramit Sethi
◆ *Killing Sacred Cows* by Garrett Gunderson
◆ *Rich Dad Poor Dad* by Robert Kiyosaki

Relational challenges can include spousal communication issues, handling your children's needs daily, or taking care of a loved one whose health is declining. These can all have deleterious effects on our well-being if they are not managed effectively. I experience some of these relational challenges and do my best to make them into positives and eustress. I am the coach for my six-year-old's T-ball team, and I am the current desired parent at bedtime for the two-year-old. At the same time, my parents, who are both retired, are taking care of my grandmother at home as she completes her ninth decade of life.

Challenges that involve love relationships can be particularly difficult as they involve our emotions. We are at our most vulnerable in these relationships, and poor communication or negative-directed energy can play a particularly devastating role on our stress levels. We can feel ecstatic when we first find someone who seems like they click with us—it's often the only thing we can think about for the first few months—while it can feel like a knife to the chest when we are in a fight, feel betrayed, or when a relationship doesn't work out. How we manage these emotions is what dictates whether something is a positive or negative—eustress or distress. Here are a couple of my favorite books on relationships and parenting:

- *Men Are from Mars, Women Are from Venus* by John Gray
- *The Conscious Parent* by Shefali Tsabary
- *The Way of the Superior Man* by David Deida (for the men)

Work or business stress can vary as well. I have clients who work in landscaping, outside daily, working long hours with physical challenges, which is very different from other clients of mine who run hedge funds, working in an office environment most of the day. The daily stress can come from commuting to work, being challenged by coworkers, and tasks that may not be completed to the level you would like, or not knowing who your next client will be.

Choosing to see these daily challenges as helping you move toward a positive goal in your life will help to shift the conversation in your head. This will allow you to begin seeing these challenges as eustress rather than distress.

CHAPTER 3

PSYCHOLOGICAL STRESSORS

This next umbrella of stressors has to do with trauma and childhood challenges. Within this bucket of psychological stress are potential triggers and issues that I like to say scuff and scratch the lenses through which we see the world. There are two major buckets here within the psychological stress section that need to be looked at with a certain amount of depth: adverse childhood events (ACEs) and major traumatic events.

Prior to age six, it has been discovered, our minds are functioning without a true sense of "self." Our parents, siblings, and nearby loved ones are simply an extension of ourselves during these early stages of life. I am watching along currently as my eldest daughter turns six years old and seeing how she has begun to separate herself and acting in a way that is focused on taking care of herself. It is a progressive change that occurs, but most parents who have watched this process will attest that there absolutely is a shift that takes place between the ages of five to eight years, when children become more independent and far more capable of taking care of themselves.

In the first four to five years of life, we are developing an understanding of the world we live in, our relationship to those around us, and basically, the way society and social dynamic works. During this time, we are building our subconscious—the part of our conscious mind that we are mostly unaware of. This explains why most people don't have a conscious memory of their lives prior to age four, as well as why we are unaware of this part of our mind and thus have created subconscious beliefs about safety, comfort, wants, needs, etc. The shift begins to happen around age four to six, when we begin to identify as ourselves and an individual.

The incidents that happen between birth and age six have a profound effect on our belief systems and how we view the world as we grow into independent and high-functioning adults. These events shape and mold our view of the world. They can often scuff or scratch the lenses through which we see the world and how we react or respond to similar or triggering incidents as functioning adults. Adverse events that take place in the first six years of our lives are often major triggers for mental health challenges, and they can often be the explanation for why we have negative or overly emotional reactions when certain topics come up in conversation.

The role of the subconscious mind is to keep you *safe*. Incidents in your childhood that made you feel *unsafe* are often the trigger for emotional dysregulation and negative habits that we implement in our lives, even though we logically know better. If finances were a trigger for your parents, and as a child you felt unsafe when you asked for a toy or for food, then this can create a trigger for you as a child. Every time finances or financial struggle are brought up by your spouse, you may feel unsafe and will compensate for the unsafe feelings by raising your voice, avoiding the subject, or doing something to raise your dopamine such as walking over to the fridge to put something tasty in your mouth, regardless of your hunger level.

Safety is the foundation of the polyvagal theory, a defining and groundbreaking explanation first presented by Dr. Stephen Porges. Dr. Porges postulates that the brain stem is the filtering point that determines which areas of the brain we will have access to, based on the state that our body is in. If we are in safe spaces, we will be able to access higher cortical functions—executive function, reasoning, and the prefrontal cortex. If we are in danger states, the activation of the brain stem will only allow access to primitive defense systems—the reptilian brain that puts up a barrier when we feel challenged, mobilizing the sympathetic nervous system—thus fight or flight.[1]

The polyvagal theory is unique because in addition to the experience of safe spaces driving parasympathetic and higher cortical functioning, and danger states driving the sympathetic activation that triggers the fight/flight response, there is a third branch that triggers a *freeze* response. This occurs when we are in an acute, very high-stress situation in which we are unable to fight or flee from the threat. This type of situation triggers a shutdown circuit, which includes a second level of defense. When a person is in a freeze response, they are simply attempting to stay alive.

Only cues of safety can help move a person out of this state, and it cannot be forced. Physiological cues of slower breathing, greater intonation in one's voice, and sounds that one can associate with safety must be employed—we will discuss these prompts and strategies in Section 3.

Psychological stressors are the first to form and the most consequential type of stressor, as these challenges arise concurrently with the development of our subconscious mind and the emotional regulation centers of the brain—the amygdala and hypothalamus. These responses are learned, and these particular circuits are formed during the highly neuroplastic development of childhood and our younger lives. This explains the physiological responses that we can have when we feel in danger or under threats as an adult, when the threats mimic those of our childhood, leading to activation of the shutdown circuit and the freeze response.

A childhood filled with safety and security will often result in a well-adjusted, higher functioning individual in most circumstances, as the neural circuits to prompt safety and higher cortical functions are strongly developed. A childhood filled with danger experiences and negative emotions will often result in an adult who is primed toward sympathetic activation as the neural circuits developed push toward a fight-or-flight style of response more readily. This will prompt physiological responses that are consistent with dysfunction and disease.

Psychological stressors, particularly during childhood but also during traumatic incidents later in life, can damage the lenses through which we see the world. They can prime us toward a sympathetic response, and this explains how some people can handle higher stress levels than others. This is a very important part of the stress bucket, and it often accounts for the foundation of the size of the bucket as well as the first part of the bucket to fill up.

To address the psychological stressor, it is important to begin asking ourselves the following question: What story am I telling myself about this situation? What is the story I'm making up in my head regarding this situation that is making me feel this way?

CHAPTER 4

PHYSICAL STRESSORS

Physical stressors are, in my opinion, a common missing piece to the puzzle of stressors that we encounter in our lives. It is an interesting piece, because this is one area that you can potentially overdo or completely miss out on.

Physical stress involves any challenge to our physical body that stops us from being able to move optimally and support our muscular and skeletal health. What's unique about physical stress is that underutilization is more of an issue than overutilization, particularly in our convenience-driven, relatively sedentary lives.

Movement is paramount for life to exist. Even the plant kingdom follows this rule of life. Plant "heliotropism" is the name we have given to plants that orient their flowers or leaves toward the sun at various times of the day. Sunflowers move their faces to the sun throughout the day, while other plant varieties will face their leaves toward either the morning sun or midday sun to optimize for sunlight exposure and maximum photosynthesis.

In the same way, humans are meant to spend time outdoors—in the sunlight. Most of us don't get outdoors and don't move enough to generate and utilize energy effectively. A sedentary life has been proven to be a precursor to each of the most common causes of disease and mortality—cardiovascular disease, cancer, and metabolic diseases.

When we don't move enough, we don't provide our muscles with a reason to function effectively. Ineffective movement leads to loss of muscle size and strength, and this is particularly evident after the age of 40, in which it has been well documented that humans will lose between 1–3 percent of their lean muscle mass per year and between 3–10 percent of their muscle strength each year.

Muscle is the organ of longevity. Dr. Gabrielle Lyon, the founder of The Center for Muscle-Centric Medicine and author of the book *Forever Strong*, is the primary proponent of this concept, and she shares that the research is very clear on this point. Muscle is an incredibly important endocrine organ and the most effective cell type at balancing insulin and blood sugar levels. Dysfunctional insulin and glucose metabolism are often at the root of chronic disease and health conditions. As we age, it is more likely that we will begin to lose muscle at an accelerated rate, which is why it is so important that we maintain healthy movement throughout our lives. Muscle loss is not a foregone conclusion and can be rebuilt on an individual basis—so let this be your motivation to get up and get moving.

You don't need to become an elite cross fitter or bodybuilder, and in fact physical stressors have a different effect on athletes (overuse and injury). Walking for 30 minutes three to five times per week has been shown to be infinitely valuable. Body-weight training without extra weight is one of the best tools that we all have access to and is highly effective in slowing muscle loss. The key takeaway is that a sedentary life is harmful to your health and a major source of distress, while some movement daily is necessary for maintaining muscle mass and supporting longevity.

On the opposite side of this coin is physical overexertion.

Athletes and weekend warriors have a tendency to overdo it and often forget about the recovery time that is necessary following a sporting event. This doesn't mean that athletics is a harmful endeavor at all, just that recovery is often overlooked and is a necessary tool in allowing the body to rebuild effectively following the stressor of movement.

After cycling from Toronto to Niagara Falls (a 140-km/90-mile challenge I have so far completed twice in my life with some wonderful friends), I took a couple of days to recuperate and allow my body to handle the recovery process as I inevitably caused some muscle breakdown, depleting nutrients and electrolytes in the process. A shorter and slower recovery ride after two or three days was the extent of my training for the next week or so following this challenge.

This is also important in the acute stages of training, as a rest time of between 60–180 seconds is required between sets of a weight-training regimen. Stretching and cryotherapy are necessary following a sporting event. During the performance of these tasks, we actually are causing rapid breakdown of muscle tissue and utilization of both macro- and micronutrients. This inevitably results in the production of by-products of cellular metabolism that need to be cleared out, biotransformed, and detoxified from the body. This can only happen when we activate the mechanisms of recovery and shift to a parasympathetic state following the performance of stated activities. Breathing is key to this state shift and is one of the main avenues we will discuss in later chapters.

Physical traumas are another important area within the physical stress section that need to be addressed. These are heavily overlooked when it comes to the timeline of chronic disease.

Concussion and traumatic brain injury (TBI), as well as automobile accidents, surgeries, and blunt- or sharp-force trauma, are all major sources of physical stress. Injuries such as these push our bodies into a sympathetic state more readily and can significantly slow the recovery process because of the sheer amount of inflammation they produce. Due to the acute and significant nature of these stressors, they can fill the proverbial stress bucket quite rapidly.

The mechanism by which concussion/TBI affects the autonomic nervous system, specifically the parasympathetic branch and vagus nerve, is through the shearing forces that damage the axons of cells extending from the brain stem, particularly those extending from the nucleus tractus solitarius (NTS). NTS is the primary afferent nucleus of the vagus nerve in the brain stem, through which signals from the peripheral organs enter the CNS, providing information on inflammation and organ function.

The axons extending from NTS are particularly susceptible to a head or whiplash type of injury, as the force of the head being propelled in nearly any direction is countered by the body compensating and attempting to hold the position it is already in. The opposition of the acceleration-deceleration force of the head moving in one direction while the body tries to hold its current position creates a vulnerability at the brain stem and spinal cord. The weight of the head makes the upper cervical and brain stem the most vulnerable to these opposing forces. This leads to a shearing force at this level, which is likely to cause diffuse axonal injury, a slicing through the longest part of the neuron, resulting in its inability to send neural signals.

Diffuse axonal injury has been found to be present in 56 percent of moderate TBI cases and 90 percent of severe TBI patients. It is very clear that any history of TBI or concussion must be considered as a potential trigger or root cause in the pathogenesis of vagus nerve dysfunction and the inability to control inflammation following this type of injury. It's particularly important to note that these injuries do not have to be recent... the more recent the injury, the more likely it is linked to the acute ability to handle inflammation; however, significant injuries of axonal damage can result in these issues slowly encroaching on the quality of life of someone who is suffering from a chronic inflammatory condition.

The name of the game when it comes to physical trauma is resilience and recovery. Recovery from these physical traumas is slower in individuals who are sedentary or have lower lean body mass and poor movement patterns. This is all the more reason to keep relatively good movement patterns and muscle strength, as these are important tools in the resilience of our bodies.

The final area of physical stress that truly matters to the state of stress on the body is the physical and mechanical function of breathing. On average, we take well over 21,000 breaths each day, but the range of this can be anywhere from 12,000 in someone with very efficient breathing patterns to over 30,000 breaths per day in those with dysfunctional breathing patterns. The mechanics of an effective breathing pattern are essential to shifting our state between parasympathetic and sympathetic. Most importantly, the vast majority of people, particularly those who suffer from chronic health conditions, are not breathing correctly, efficiently, or effectively.

There are three physical areas that need to be addressed when it comes to the physical stress of improper breathing patterns—the first is the nasal passage, the second is the mouth/oral cavity, and the third is the diaphragm.

The nasal passage is our primary breathing tube. We evolved to have nasal hairs present at the opening of this passage, which act as a physical filter to particulate matter and potential allergens floating in the air. We don't have nose hairs in our mouth, and we don't have teeth in our nose. The nose is the breathing tube and the mouth is the eating tube. It's great to have a backup pathway should the nasal passage become blocked or physically incapable of having air pass through it for various reasons, and that is what the mouth is very useful for.

Breathing through the nose helps to slow the breath rate, which is the most effective way to shift our state to parasympathetic. If we do not require high quantities of oxygen because we are not performing a physically demanding task, nasal breathing is great to keep the breath rate down and help activate the vagus nerve, keeping us in a rest/digest/recover state. Physical blockage or inefficiency of the nasal passage plays a significant role in pushing our state toward sympathetic fight/flight.

The most common reasons for inefficient nasal breathing are a deviated septum and sinus blockages, both challenges that I have personally dealt with. A deviated septum is particularly challenging to overcome as it results from less than optimal physical development of bone and cartilage making up the nasal septum. This can happen due to physical trauma (I broke my nose at age four when I was hit square in the face by a baseball bat) and also due to chronically poor tongue positioning during passive nasal breathing.

Tongue position is particularly overlooked and missed — so it should be at the forefront of your mind if you happen to breathe through your mouth. When we are relaxed or calm, 100 percent of our breathing should happen through our nose. During this time, the top of the tongue should actually be placed on the front of our hard palate, just behind our upper incisors on the midline. The nasal septum is calcified and formed throughout the first 12 years of life, based on the pressure of the tongue resting on the roof of the oral cavity. This is especially true while we are sleeping, as we are generally not eating, talking, or exercising while we are asleep. Ideally, our tongue rests with a mild amount of pressure on the palate or roof of our mouths, forcing us to breathe through our nose. A deviated septum is highly correlated to mouth breathing during childhood and is particularly challenging to overcome as an adult without surgical intervention.

Sinus blockage can actually occur secondarily to a deviated septum but is highly correlated to mouth breathing as well. Just as air passage through the oral cavity leads to a dry mouth, air passage through the nose decreases sinus congestion and blockage. In a vicious cycle, mouth breathing causes sinus congestion and thus a blocked nasal passage, resulting in required breathing through the mouth. This is a difficult cycle to overcome and requires active attention to your breathing pattern and making regular changes. Once you begin breathing through your nose more regularly, sinus congestion will decrease significantly, but the initial changes need to be active rather than passive.

The diaphragm is the primary muscle of breathing but tends to be underutilized in most people. Most of us actually use secondary breathing muscles more than the diaphragm to drive our breath. The secondary breathing muscles are the intercostal muscles located between each of the ribs, the trapezius (aka "traps") and rhomboids between the shoulder and upper back, and the muscles connecting the spine to the ribs, known as the "scalenes." When these secondary muscles are overused, they result in shorter, shallower breaths as well as tighter muscles in the neck and upper back.

A simple test to see which muscles you are currently using is to do the following: Put one hand on your upper chest and the other hand on your belly. Close your eyes and take a normal breath. Feel which hand is moving with your inhale and exhale. If the hand on your chest is moving forward with your inhale, then you are using your accessory breathing muscles more readily and are shifting your state toward sympathetic. If the hand on your belly is moving more, then the diaphragm is being used more readily and your state is shifting toward parasympathetic. This is a test you can utilize at any time to help you become more mindful of your current breath pattern and autonomic state. You can consciously focus on shifting your breath to the diaphragm and breathe through the nose to help shift your state upon using this test.

Ineffective breathing mechanics are a direct physical stressor and one that we most certainly overlook. Your goal regarding breathing should be to focus on slower, nasal, and diaphragmatic breath, and we will discuss specific breathing exercises in later chapters to give you practices that you can implement immediately.

CHAPTER 5

BIOCHEMICAL STRESSORS

The final category of stressors that we will address are the biochemical stressors, and this is the form of stress that has come into the limelight over the past 10–15 years with the ever-increasing use of chemicals and plastics, the extensive research into the microbiome, significant improvements in understanding nutrition, and learning more about how technology and various radio and electromagnetic frequencies can affect our biology. In this section, we will dig into some of the more well-researched forms of biochemical stress that affect the vagus nerve, causing our bodies to remain chronically in a state of sympathetic activation.

NUTRITION AND MITOCHONDRIAL FUNCTION

There are two very particular areas to cover here within the nutrition component of biochemical stress affecting the vagus nerve. First are the nutrients that we need, though many people are deficient, and second are the dietary choices that cause distress to our cellular, inflammatory, and overall body systems.

The vagus nerve utilizes acetylcholine as its only neurotransmitter—the chemical messenger that relays the message from one nerve cell to any other type of cell. Acetylcholine is used throughout the body for various other processes, most importantly nerve control of muscle function and regulation of immune cells.

Acetylcholine is built in our body from two parts: acetyl-CoA and choline.

Acetyl-CoA is a very important molecule in the production of cellular energy in the mitochondria. Every cell in our body contains mitochondria, the "powerhouse" or "battery" of the cell. The role of mitochondria is to produce cellular energy, known as ATP or adenosine triphosphate—an adenosine molecule attached to three phosphate groups. The bonds of each phosphate contain a high amount of potential energy, and when one of these bonds is broken (ATP = ADP + P), it releases energy by which the cell is able to carry out its important role in the body. Without ATP, cells cannot complete their particular role.

Essential to the production of ATP are carbohydrates (glucose) and fats (triglycerides and fatty acids). Glucose goes through a process called "glycolysis" in the cytoplasm of the cell, during which it is broken down from a six-carbon molecule into two three-carbon molecules known as "pyruvic acid" or "pyruvate." Pyruvate is then moved into the mitochondria, where it is converted into the substrate acetyl-CoA.

Acetyl-CoA has multiple roles in the cell. The first is to enter and begin a process in the mitochondria known as the "Krebs cycle" or "citric acid cycle." This process is meant to produce high amounts of NADH and FADH2; these two molecules then enter the electron transport chain to create ATP. The second function of acetyl-CoA is to exit the mitochondria and become the first part of the molecule in question here—acetylcholine.

The process of glycolysis (glucose → pyruvate → acetyl-CoA) requires some very important micronutrients—vitamins B1 and B3, chromium, lipoic acid, and CoQ10 are at the top of this list. Diets lacking these nutrients will reduce the efficacy by which the breakdown of glucose can occur. The decreased ability to break down glucose over a longer timeline will likely result in insulin resistance, a major stressor to the body, as well as reduced production of acetyl-CoA.

Acetyl-CoA is also produced from the breakdown of fatty acids, glycerol, and cholesterol. Once our body has digested fatty acids via the gut or extracted them from adipose cells, the free fatty acids must be used up in order to avoid triggering an inflammatory process in the circulatory system. We can utilize the fatty acids to produce acetyl-CoA in the mitochondria. Upon taking a lipoprotein (a transport molecule that contains fatty acids or cholesterol) into the cell, we need to transport the fatty acid into the mitochondria, a process that requires a nutrient called "carnitine."

In order to move fatty acids into the mitochondria, we require the carnitine shuttle to be functioning well. The carnitine shuttle requires that our cells contain an optimal level of carnitine to be present, as well as butyrate, a by-product of symbiotic intestinal bacteria to facilitate the process.

Carnitine can itself be produced within the body, but dietary sources help to ensure that our levels are optimal. The best dietary sources of carnitine include beef, pork, poultry and dairy products. We will discuss butyrate in the next subsection related to the microbiome and optimal gut function.

Once enough acetyl-CoA is produced to enter the Krebs cycle and facilitate mitochondrial production of ATP, a percentage of it exits the mitochondria and prepares to be connected to choline to produce the neurotransmitter acetylcholine.

Deficiency of B vitamins and many of these important nutrients is a rampant issue in diets focused on ultraprocessed convenience foods. When these important nutrients are lacking from dietary sources and are unable to be utilized effectively due to limited movement and poor muscle cell quality, the result is mitochondrial dysfunction. Dysfunctional mitochondria constitute a major step in the inflammatory cascade leading to premature cell death and disease. This will also result in a reduced capacity to produce acetyl-CoA and thus acetylcholine (ACh). Lack of ACh will then lead to poor signaling capacity of the vagus nerve among other nerves and cells that utilize ACh as their main signaling molecule.

CHOLINE DEFICIENCY

Choline, the second molecule required to produce ACh, follows a much simpler route to the cell. It is an essential dietary nutrient, meaning that we cannot produce choline in our cells; we must take it in from our dietary or supplemental sources.

The issue that occurs in this situation is that as a species, we are chronically deficient in this important nutrient. Multiple studies have concluded that approximately 90 percent of North Americans are deficient in choline intake and choline levels in the body.

Choline enters the bloodstream through the gut and is taken up into the cells via a choline and sodium (Na+) transporter, meaning that we also require sodium to be able to transport choline into the cell, where it can be combined with acetyl-CoA to finally produce

ACh. Sodium is most commonly brought into the body via salt and other electrolyte sources.

There are a few different supplemental sources of choline, all with similar absorption rates, but with differing bacterial metabolism rates. Choline bitartrate, choline chloride, alpha-glycerophosphorylcholine (alpha-GPC), and phosphatidylcholine are all forms of choline that can be supplemented. For all four forms, the choline levels in the bloodstream increase within two to six hours at very similar rates, and all will decline quite rapidly following the six-hour mark.

Where these four forms of choline supplementation differ is in bacterial metabolism and the production of the bacterial metabolite trimethylamine N-oxide (TMAO). TMAO has been linked to a higher risk of cardiovascular disease, not as a causative issue, but higher TMAO derived from bacterial metabolism is linked to cholesterol metabolism alterations, inflammatory cytokine levels, endothelial dysfunction in the blood vessels, and platelet activation. Higher levels of TMAO may not cause cardiovascular disease, but they are clearly associated.[2]

Choline bitartrate and choline chloride, the salt forms of choline, were found to be associated with higher levels of TMAO following intake. Alpha-GPC did show slight elevations in TMAO, but of the supplemental forms, it had the smallest increase. Dietary source phosphatidylcholine from eggs was found to have almost zero increase in TMAO levels, showing that this particular dietary source seems to be the best option for ensuring lower TMAO levels.[3]

Adult males require a minimum of 550 mg/day of choline, while females require between 400–425mg/day. The top 11 best dietary sources of choline are as follows:

TOP 11 BEST DIETARY SOURCES OF CHOLINE*

Food Source	Milligrams (mg per serving)	Percent DV
Beef liver, pan fried, 3 ounces	356	65
Egg, hard boiled, 1 large egg	147	27
Beef top round, separable lean only, braised, 3 ounces	117	21
Soybeans, roasted, ½ cup	107	19
Chicken breast, roasted, 3 ounces	72	13
Beef, ground, 93 percent lean meat, broiled, 3 ounces	72	13
Fish, cod, Atlantic, cooked, dry heat, 3 ounces	71	13
Potatoes, red, baked, flesh and skin, 1 large potato	57	10
Wheat germ, toasted, 1 ounce	51	9
Beans, kidney, canned, ½ cup	45	8
Quinoa, cooked, 1 cup	43	8

* Source: https://ods.od.nih.gov/factsheets/Choline-HealthProfessional

It is very clear that the production of acetyl-CoA and the presence of choline are absolutely necessary for optimal vagus nerve function, and deficiencies in either or in the cofactors that support the production of these nutrients are a stressor that are likely holding back vagus nerve health.

Take some time to assess your diet, nutrition, and supplement status to determine if this is a challenge for you or if your nutrition could be better, and then attempt to improve your overall nutrient status. My favorite nutrition-tracking app is called Cronometer (no affiliation) because it is customizable to your dietary and macronutrient preferences, but it's also a great tracker of specific micronutrients, amino acids, and other essential nutrients for optimal health.

PRODUCTION OF ACETYLCHOLINE

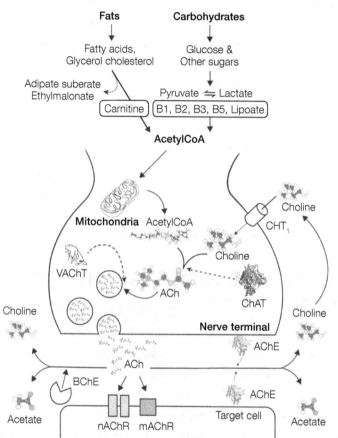

This image shows the biochemical pathways involved in the production of acetylcholine. In the mitochondria, dietary fats are effectively broken down to acetyl-CoA in the presence of carnitine, while dietary carbohydrates follow the pyruvate-lactate pathway to produce acetyl-CoA in the presence of B-vitamins and lipoic acid.

Choline and acetyl-CoA are paired together to produce acetylcholine, which is released into the synapse and binds to the acetylcholine receptors on the target cells, which can include other neurons and immune cells, among others.

DIETARY SOURCES OF BIOCHEMICAL STRESS

Our diet is one of the most common sources of biochemical stress and triggers for inflammation. The Standard American Diet (appropriately known as SAD) is built on the basis of convenience and hyperpalatability. What this means is that the foods that are most commonly consumed by the North American population (although this diet is quickly becoming the standard worldwide diet) is high in calories, low in nutrient density, and heavily processed with the intent of driving dopamine levels up in our brains.

Going through all of the sources of inflammation in our diets would require an additional 50,000 words in this book, so I will go over the top five most common culprits in driving biochemical stress and inflammation from a dietary perspective.

1. SUGAR AND HIGH-CARBOHYDRATE DIETS

One of the most significant challenges of the past four to five decades is sugar and hidden sources of simple carbohydrates. As the agricultural industry has shifted to monocropping and higher yield foods such as corn and soy, the food industry has tried to make the foods they produce more palatable. The effect of this with regard to our biochemistry has been heavily processed foods that drive a strong dopamine response. Sugar and high-fructose corn syrup are at the root of this trend toward hyperpalatability.

As the human population grew significantly after the Second World War, the need to feed all these people has slowly but very clearly led to the production of foods and food products that don't spoil as quickly, are more convenient to travel with, are easier to

UPGRADE YOUR VAGUS NERVE

store in our homes, and still taste good. Initially the trend in this direction was slow, but as our lives became faster paced, the desire for convenience has increased drastically.

Humans, like all animals, are wired to eat what tastes good and drives a fulfillment response. A good taste in our mouths is a sign that we are receiving energy-rich and nutrient-dense foods. Unfortunately, this physiological response has been hijacked by the food industry. Foods that we used to eat that were both higher in energy (calories) and nutrients (micro- and macronutrients) are more difficult to farm and get into everyone's hands. The food industry began to create foods that had longer shelf lives but still had enough caloric density to contribute to our energy needs. In doing so, nutrient density was sacrificed.

Slowly and surely, the food industry has created a narrative that the most important thing about what you eat is how it tastes, and on the health side, how many calories it contains. We have followed along with this narrative due to the dopaminergic response that we feel when we eat heavily processed, hyperpalatable, high-energy foods that unfortunately lack nutrient density.

To increase the palatability of these processed food products, sugar and refined carbohydrates have been used and are now consumed in unprecedented amounts. Estimates of individual sugar intake in the 2020s range between 57 to 180 pounds per person each year! This is a staggering statistic, but even more frightening is that sugar consumption from beet and cane sources has decreased. From 1970 to 1985, the annual consumption of corn-based sweeteners, particularly high-fructose corn syrup (HFCS), rose to contribute nearly 150 calories per day and by all metrics, HFCS is significantly more dangerous from a physiological perspective.

Since the introduction of HFCS into the human diet, rates of type 2 diabetes, obesity, fatty liver disease, cancer, and chronic inflammatory health conditions have skyrocketed. The ability of our bodies to effectively metabolize sugar and HFCS has been steadily decreasing as we have also become more sedentary, sitting at our desks, on our couches, and in our cars for between 6 and 15 hours each day. Our ability to utilize the increasing quantity of calories that we are taking in has been compromised by our decreasing muscle mass and movement patterns.

Excessive intake of sugars and HFCS has been closely linked to the development of many chronic health conditions. In an article by Ma, et al. in *Frontiers in Immunology* in August 2022, they linked the excessive intake of sugar to multiple sclerosis, rheumatoid arthritis, psoriasis, and inflammatory bowel disease.[4] They clearly discussed the association between excessive sugar consumption and intestinal permeability (also known as "leaky gut syndrome"). In a study by Jameel et al., they compared the effects of fructose, glucose, and sucrose on blood levels of LDL, HDL, and triglycerides with regard to blood lipids, and hs-CRP, a very sensitive biomarker of inflammation in the body. What was special about this study is that it was completed in a healthy population. What they found was very revealing—fructose consumption (in the form of fructose-infused sugary drinks with 50 g fructose taken in a fasting state, not directly from fruit sources, which contain significantly less fructose and many other nutrients necessary for optimal functioning) was responsible for directly increasing total cholesterol, LDL, HDL, and hs-CRP values significantly more than glucose and fructose at 30 and 60 minutes post-consumption. Glucose and sucrose were both triggers for significantly elevated triglyceride levels.[5]

Jameel et al. concluded that fructose consumption in the form of HFCS-containing sugary drinks was responsible for major inflammatory and cholesterol changes in the acute phase. We can infer from this that the continued consumption of drinks containing HFCS (those that lack any of the beneficial nutrients from proper fruit consumption) is detrimental to our health by the direct changes to inflammatory and cholesterol levels in the body.

By damaging the gut lining and causing a leaky gut, sugar enables the elevation of LPS and other inflammatory triggers to enter the body and signal the immune cells of the gut and the rest of the body to initiate the inflammatory cascade. Sugar consumption is linked directly to activation of the NF-kB and JAK2/STAT3 pathways, which increase the expression of inflammatory cytokines. It is also directly linked to mitochondrial release of reactive oxygen species (ROS), which leads to cellular and DNA damage, exasperating the inflammatory cascade.

Put these conditions together and you create metabolic dysfunction, and inflammation triggers that push on the aforementioned accelerator pedal, activating the sympathetic nervous system. Poor glucose metabolism from sugar and HFCS intake are major contributors to the biochemical stress pathway. They are, however, a relatively simple area for positive change for those who want to take action.

2. INFLAMMATORY SEED OILS (HIGH OMEGA-6 FATS)

It would be a disservice to focus on sugars as the only dietary source of inflammation as more research emerges on the inflammatory effects of seed oils that are prevalent and relatively hidden in our conventional diets.

Fats are one of the three macronutrients that our body requires (in addition to carbohydrates and protein), and they can be derived from many natural sources. Traditionally and in many older cultures, fats come from dairy sources (butter, ghee, cream), egg yolks, olive, avocado and some other fruits, and all meat sources. These are some of the healthiest forms of fats that we can have in our diets.

Over the past 50 years, the cost of obtaining these fat sources increased significantly, leading to industrial innovation to find newer and less expensive sources of fats. As revolutionary as this sounds, it seems to have come at a significant cost to our health, as many of these previously alternative sources contain a very high ratio of omega-6 fatty acids compared to the healthier and less inflammatory omega-3 fatty acids present in higher quantities in healthier fats. Even more significant is how these oils are sourced and processed.

These newer sources include vegetable and industrial seed oils such as soybean, canola, corn, safflower, and sunflower oils, which are very high in linoleic acid. Soybean oil makes up nearly 20 percent of all calories consumed in the United States, which is an astounding figure due to its very high omega-6 to omega-3 ratio. Excess omega-6 consumption is clearly an inflammatory trigger affecting blood vessels and sparking the inflammatory cascade, as it breaks down to arachidonic acid, which competes with EPA and DHA from omega-3 sources.

Oils high in polyunsaturated fat, particularly omega-6 polyunsaturated fatty acids (PUFAs), are ultimately the fat source to avoid. The eight types of oils to try to avoid are canola, corn, cottonseed, soybean, sunflower, safflower, grape seed, and rice-bran oil. Be very cognizant of these oils when looking at the ingredient lists present on your food choices, and I highly recommend eliminating all of these oils for cooking. Stick to grass-fed butter, ghee, beef tallow, olive oil, coconut oil, and avocado oil.

3. INSUFFICIENT PROTEIN INTAKE

Continuing the discussion on macronutrients, we come to the most important macronutrient of all—which just so happens to be the one that most people are not getting sufficient amounts of in their daily diet—protein.

Amino acids are the building blocks of our body—I like to refer to them as the Lego blocks that we can use to create proteins of varying shapes, sizes, and configurations, each with a very different but important function within the body.

The most abundant protein in the human body is collagen, with seven different forms of collagen that our bodies use as the glue that literally holds us together. This includes skin, muscle, fascia, connective tissue, and blood vessels holding each of our organs in their correct anatomical location.

Muscle tissue is the greatest source of amino acid storage within the body, and as was discussed previously, muscle loss accelerates as we age. On an average basis, humans will lose between 1–3 percent of muscle mass each year after age 40. This muscle loss is actually caused by breakdown and loss of stored protein within the body.

If our protein intake and movement levels (muscle use) are not sufficient, our body needs to break down the muscle to make amino acids available for proper cellular function and processes. This is a catabolic process, meaning a breakdown of a source of raw materials to make the components available for other sources. Catabolic processes are a normal homeostatic function, but they happen primarily when raw materials are scarce and hard to come across.

As we age and our protein intake seems insufficient while our movement patterns and muscle use are less than optimal due to a sedentary lifestyle, this accelerates the catabolic process of muscular breakdown. Accelerated breakdown of muscle is a dysfunctional state; however, a major sign of full disease state is known as "cachexia," which is severe muscle loss that is common in cancer and severe autoimmune disease.

The catabolic signaling to break down muscles is actually an inflammatory process, mediated by the innate immune cells in the muscle tissue—a very important topic that we will come back to when discussing tissue-resident macrophages and the cholinergic anti-inflammatory pathway.

In order to avoid the accelerated breakdown of muscle tissue, there are two things we can do—take in sufficient quantities of protein on a daily basis and keep using our muscles as much as possible with daily movement. With muscle, the concept of "if you don't use it, you'll lose it" is entirely accurate. This is a concept that should drive home the idea of building muscle and moving daily to ensure you don't lose muscle.

Regarding protein intake, here are some simple-to-follow guidelines:

Activity Level	Recommendation (g protein/kg ideal weight)	Example (Person Who Is 150 lbs/68 kg)
Base Requirements	0.8–1.2 g/kg	54–81 g daily
Recreationally Active	1.4–1.8 g/kg	95–122 g daily
Endurance Athletes	1.8–2.0 g/kg	122–136 g daily
Strength Athletes	2.0–2.2 g/kg	136–150 g daily

4. SNACKING AND LATE-NIGHT EATING

One area that many of us struggle with, myself included, concerns snacking and late-night eating. The challenge here is that food eaten at less-than-optimal times can be dysregulating to the hormonal system within the body.

Insulin is our body's master hormone for the regulation of blood sugar levels. When we eat, particularly the consumption of carbohydrate-containing foods, our blood sugar levels will rise after the carbs are digested and absorbed from the intestinal tract. In response to the increase in blood glucose, the pancreas is signaled to release insulin into the bloodstream as well.

The effect of insulin is to increase glucose transport from the blood into all cells of the body. Insulin binds to the insulin receptors on the surface of most cells, triggering glucose transportation via facilitated diffusion into the cells to be used for the production of cellular energy via glycolysis (remember glucose → acetyl-CoA). The acetyl-CoA can then be input into the mitochondria to undergo transformation in the Krebs cycle and electron transport chain to produce cellular energy in the form of ATP. The cells that are most efficient at this are liver cells, muscle cells, and adipose (fat storage) cells.

In the liver, glucose is absorbed and converted into a storage form called "glycogen." Glycogen is stored in the liver until it is needed to support an increase in blood sugar in the body when the energy needs are greater than the supply in the blood—this happens most commonly during exercise. Muscle cells use glucose very effectively when we move a lot, and this can lower the amount of circulating sugars, so the liver sends glucose out to increase the amount of circulating glucose. This results in depletion of glycogen stores within the liver. To replete glycogen storage, the liver is the first place that glucose goes when we take in carbs and blood sugar levels are sufficient. But when the glycogen stores are full, the liver will stop accepting glucose. Then the muscle and adipose cells become the prime acceptors of glucose from the bloodstream.

In my previous book, we discussed the issues of insulin resistance and how this is a major biochemical stressor in the body. Insulin is a very important hormone, but one that the cells will only answer the door for if the cell itself has a need for energy production at the time that insulin comes knocking. The concept of insulin resistance is paramount to the understanding of homeostasis and energy regulation. It is of particular importance now due to the increased rate of diagnosis of metabolic syndromes, type 2 diabetes, Alzheimer's disease, obesity, and cardiovascular disease.

The more often that insulin levels spike, the more often it is knocking on the door of each cell to take in glucose and produce ATP. If blood sugar spikes are happening five to eight times per day, insulin spikes will follow and will knock on the doors of the cells five to eight times per day. This can become annoying and challenging for the cells to manage as they are being asked to take in a lot of glucose. If the cells are not in need of more energy, they will stop answering the door when insulin comes knocking.

At the cellular level, this means putting fewer and fewer insulin receptors on the surface of the cells. This results in cells not answering the door for insulin and glucose to enter. Slowly and surely, the result is increased blood glucose levels and the pancreas pushing out higher quantities of insulin to try to lower and regulate the blood sugar levels.

There are certain cell types that are willing to accept the glucose—adipose cells, or fat cells. As mentioned, these adipose cells are fat storage cells. They take in the glucose and convert it to G-6-phosphate and then to storage forms of fats called "triglycerides." The more sugars we ask our adipose cells to store, the greater the size and quantity of these adipose cells, which results in weight gain via increases in body fat levels. There are genetic variances in the quantity and size of adipose cells. Some people are genetically predisposed to having a smaller quantity of cells, and thus the size of these cells can increase drastically. Others have no such predisposition and can have a virtually unlimited number of adipose cells form in their body, which allows the size of each cell to remain smaller. The size of adipocytes is important when it comes to triggering inflammatory processes—a concept we will explore in the next section.

Chronically high levels of insulin and the cumulative effects of repeated insulin spikes are a trigger that predisposes innate immune cells toward an inflammatory signature. The innate immune cells involved in this are called "macrophages" and are the most important cell type when it comes to inflammatory control within the body. Macrophages can be found in nearly every tissue and are the main assessor of regulatory status and threats to optimal function within these tissues.

Macrophages will be a major topic in the next section of this book. For now, simply note the following: Macrophages shift states between a controlled anti-inflammatory state and an uncontrolled inflammatory state. Hyperinsulinemia (high levels of insulin in the blood) is a trigger to push macrophages into the inflammatory state, predisposing them to exaggerated levels of inflammation and hypersensitivity to other inflammatory triggers.

Control of insulin levels is an overlooked component in the inflammatory cascade and something that we need to take into account when we are addressing the dietary components of biochemical stress. Diets high in processed food, sugar, and inflammatory seed oils create an internal environment of excessive insulin and predispose us to chronic inflammatory conditions.

5. LOW ELECTROLYTE LEVELS/ DEHYDRATION

The final dietary source of biochemical stress that I would like to discuss here is one that has been missing from the discussion, as it can be perceived to be too simple. This is an issue that I have experienced quite intensely on a few occasions, particularly when I am completing physical activity over a longer period of time, specifically the loss of electrolytes due to dehydration.

When we hear the word "dehydration," we often think of low levels of water in the body. While this definition is technically true, the actual cause of lower levels of body water is not sufficiently explained by this term.

I specifically remember the moment I felt my brain start working again... I was completing a cycling training ride with a friend of mine. We were training to ride from Toronto to Niagara Falls, approximately 140 km (90 miles). This training ride was supposed to be a total of 100 km, from Toronto to Burlington and back, along the north shore of Lake Ontario. It was around the 70 km mark on our way back home that my calves began to cramp up between pedal strokes. I asked my friend to stop with me so I could stretch for a few minutes and drink some water. We were on our way back to Toronto, on a stretch of Lakeshore Road that didn't have any stores or places to stop within about 10 or 15 minutes.

We stopped and I stretched out my calves and legs, while drinking some water. A couple minutes later we got back on the bike, but my vision seemed a bit fuzzy. I could see everything, but it took me longer to process and understand exactly what I was seeing while we rode along. My speed had declined significantly, and I was laboring through the next 15 minutes of riding through some side streets. My breathing was more difficult than it had been for the previous 70 km, and my pedaling felt extremely sluggish.

We finally reached a coffee shop in Port Credit, Mississauga, and stopped for a longer break before heading home. My wonderful friend (who also happens to work as a pharmacist) ran in and got me a coconut water from the coffee shop. I began sipping it slowly—I remember the taste hitting my tongue and the immediate feeling of energy coming back into each of my muscles. After a few minutes, I felt my brain begin to turn on again. My vision became clearer, my cognition and mental processing speed returned to normal.

I soon realized that during this ride, my body was sweating quite a bit, as it was the early afternoon on a humid summer day in August in Toronto. The excessive sweating led to loss of more salt and electrolytes than I normally would lose during a workout or cycling ride. The loss of these electrolytes led to various symptoms of temporary conditions known generally as electrolyte loss—hyponatremia, hypokalemia, and hypocalcemia—severely low levels of sodium, potassium, and calcium in my body.

Electrolytes are minerals that are found in salt compounds in nature, but they break up into their ionic components when dissolved in water or in body fluids. The most simple and effective example of this is basic sea salt—sodium chloride ($NaCl$ for the science people). Sodium (Na on the periodic table) and chloride (Cl on the periodic table) are two minerals that effectively bond together to form sea salt (90 percent of sea salt is $NaCl$).

Sodium has one electron on its outer electron layer, and chloride has seven electrons on its outer layer. Minerals on Earth tend to do best with an even number of electrons in their outer layer, and when these two elements come together, sodium will share its extra electron with the seven that are on the outer layer of chloride to form a compound—NaCl—that has eight electrons in its shared outer layer, making it much more stable. When we put sea salt in water, the salt dissolves as the sodium donates its single electron to chloride, creating Na^+ and Cl^-. These charged ions then dissolve in water so that we can't visualize them anymore. The polarity between the Na^+, Cl^-, and H_2O is quite strong, as they are heavily attracted to one another. Salt dissolves in water, but water will also follow these salts and ions in their movement and directional flow.

Electrolytes are released by our sweat glands to pull out water in the form of sweat, as water follows electrolytes and salt when our internal body temperature rises. The effect of sweat evaporating from our skin is meant to extract heat and keep cooler temperatures on the body to reduce the internal body temperature. I learned the hard way exactly what can happen when you sweat out electrolytes and don't replenish them.

Our kidneys also utilize this important feature very readily to move water through the filtering process. The job of the kidney is to filter the blood to release toxins in the form of urea, another salt from the body. Urea becomes dissolved in water and is released through urination. In order to move the water through the filtering structures called "glomeruli," the kidney moves salt so that water will follow these ions, a process called "osmosis." When they are working correctly, the kidneys push out and resorb these ions through a process known as "active transportation." As you can imagine, any dysfunction to the kidney will result in the inability to filter out toxins from the blood.

The kidneys are highly effective at this process. It is a delicate balancing act for our kidneys to move salt out of the bloodstream, causing the movement of water and toxins out of the blood and into the bladder for release from the body. All mammals including humans have a similar filtering mechanism that involves a balance of water and these electrolytes. There are six main electrolytes that are essential for our optimal bodily functions: sodium, potassium, calcium, magnesium, chloride, and phosphate. Let's briefly review each of them here.

Sodium is regulated by the kidneys and is heavily involved in the removal of water and toxins. The optimal range is between 135–142 mmol/L (millimoles per liter) and any increase or decrease in salts has significant effects on brain function, like headache, nausea, restlessness, or cognitive difficulty. Hyponatremia (low sodium) is the most common electrolyte imbalance, and as such, IV fluids that are given in healthcare settings contain a higher content of sodium chloride to help restore or maintain hydration and electrolyte balance.

Potassium is used by the kidneys and in most other cells to regulate the balance of sodium (through a sodium-potassium ATP pump) and is important for energy production in the mitochondria. Optimal range of potassium is between 4.4–5.0 mmol/L. Imbalance of potassium (hyper- or hypokalemia) causes muscle cramping or generalized weakness due to its involvement in energy production.

Calcium is obviously important for the structure of bones in our bodies and is also very important in the regulation of the blood-clotting process, the polarization of neurons to transmit nerve impulses, secretion of hormones, and contraction of muscles. Optimal range for calcium levels is 9.2–10.1 mmol/L.

Chloride is most linked to sodium for intake into our bodies and is involved in processes of digestion (limiting loss of water via stool) and has been implicated in congestive heart failure.

Magnesium is highly involved in the metabolism of ATP in the muscles and brain. As such, an imbalance in magnesium levels results in a reduced capacity to use ATP as the currency of energy in the body. Symptomatically, low magnesium will result in poor cognitive function due to involvement in neurotransmitter release and overall neurological function, weak muscle contractibility, and low energy. In practice, I also notice that low magnesium levels are a trigger for poor sleep quality and even insomnia.

Eighty-five percent of the phosphorus in our bodies is stored as hydroxyapatite in our bones and teeth. Fifteen percent is involved in the metabolic function of our muscles and soft tissues. Phosphorus function usually goes hand in hand with calcium and is regulated by vitamin D3, parathyroid hormone, and calcitonin.

OPTIMAL ELECTROLYTE LEVELS ON BLOOD WORK

	Conventional Low	Optimal Low	Optimal High	Conventional High
Sodium (mmol/L)	135	135	142	145
Potassium (mmol/L)	3.6	4.4	5.0	5.5
Calcium (mg/dl)	8.8	9.2	10.1	10.7
Chloride (mmol/L)	98	100	106	110
Magnesium (mg/dl)	1.5	2.0	2.5	2.5
Phosphorus (mg/dl)	2.8	3.5	4.0	4.5

The best dietary sources of electrolytes provided by nature are fruits and vegetables with high water content: watermelon, cantaloupe, kiwi, celery, cucumber, coconut water, banana, avocado, leafy greens, and mushrooms. You can also get a lot of electrolytes from sea salt, table salt, and bone broth. For those who are exercising regularly, electrolyte-replenishing salt packets are a great option and one that I ride with or use for any exercise that I do regularly.

The importance of electrolyte balance in the optimal function of the body cannot be overstated. Mild deviations of these values over a longer period are a commonly overlooked cause of biochemical stress, so your diet and supplement protocol should involve maintaining an optimal balance in these electrolytes. Effective hydration means much more than drinking more water. I found this out the hard way. Luckily, I didn't get injured during this ride and did make it home after riding a little over 100 km with my friend. I am now quite conscious of electrolyte intake and dietary nutrient intake with every workout, especially when I plan to sweat during a workout.

MICROBIOME

One of the most common findings I see in my clients is an imbalanced microbiome. We have tens of trillions of bacteria within our gut that are working symbiotically with us. The food that we eat goes to them first—they get first choice of the nutrients that are present in the foods we consume. Depending on the balance of the population in the gut, the bacteria can work to support us or to create challenges for us when they are not working to reinforce positive choices and habits. The balance of the microbiome plays a major role in biochemical stress and is also heavily linked to metabolism, immune function, VN function, and obviously, microbiome-gut-brain axis function.

Contrary to popular belief, the presence of dysbiotic bacteria (bacteria that can be problematic if found at a high level) is actually not the most common issue I find when performing functional stool tests with my clients. The single most common issue I find is the imbalance of desirable gut bacteria called "commensal" or "keystone bacteria."

Microbiome research is constantly changing and finding new strains and new ways to assess the presence of good and less optimal species. In the past decade, there has been no greater finding than the keystone strain known as *Akkermansia muciniphila*. *Akkermansia* is a newly discovered bacterial strain that, when low, has been found to have major ties to leaky gut syndrome, metabolic conditions, and immune system dysregulation.

Akkermansia is an anaerobic gram-negative bacterium that was first discovered to be present in the human intestinal tract in 2004, and it has since become the darling of microbiome researchers. *Muciniphila* literally means "mucus loving," and this hints directly at the importance of this particular strain and its function of maintaining the layer of mucus present in front of the epithelial cells of the gut lining. This bacteria interacts with goblet cells in the lining of the gut to support their function of producing mucus as a protective barrier. The mere presence of *Akkermansia muciniphila* in the gut is a stimulant to the goblet cells to maintain a strong and protective mucus barrier. Signals from the VN are necessary to stimulate the goblet cells to produce and secrete the mucus to increase and maintain the size of the barrier, and to limit the damage of any dysbiotic bacteria. ACh is the main signal to promote the activity of goblet cells in the production of the protective mucus barrier, thus the goblet cells are reliant on both the presence of *Akkermansia* bacteria as well as effective VN inputs of ACh to create and maintain the mucosal barrier and protect against harmful microbes and certain dietary proteins.

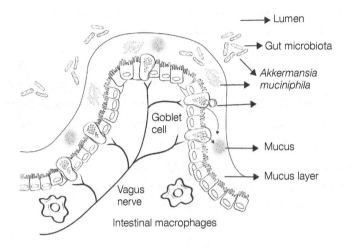

Any reduction in the size of the outer and inner layers of mucus creates conditions allowing for toxins to break down the epithelial lining of the gut, resulting in intestinal hyperpermeability, also known as "leaky gut syndrome." Leaky gut has been implicated as a causative factor in nearly all chronic health conditions, from obesity to autoimmunity. A dysfunctional gut is the most common pathway by which toxins can enter the body and trigger an inflammatory reaction, which, left unchecked over time, is the pathway to these diseases.

High levels of dysbiosis (bacterial, fungal, parasitic) or certain dietary proteins (gliadin from gluten or casein from dairy, for example) have often been cited as the cause of these chronic health conditions, but the evidence is clear that it is not simply the presence of these dysbiotic microbes or proteins that triggers conditions to occur. Certain circumstances need to be met to allow the microbes or proteins to have their biochemical stress effects. The size of the mucus barrier is directly related to this, and thus the relationship between *Akkermansia muciniphila*, vagus nerve function, and goblet cells is necessary to protect against the circumstances becoming primed for breakdown.

I have personally seen many clients experience significant, positive changes in their health status when we concurrently work on addressing microbiome factors, vagus nerve function, and dietary choices. Working to eliminate unwanted bacteria is an acceptable approach, but one should not forget to prime the gut for future potential insult or challenge. Building the mucus barrier can be beneficial to address both acute circumstances and future challenges.

TOXIC CHEMICALS AND POLLUTANTS

A litany of biochemical toxins and stressors constantly surrounds those who are living a conventional and modern lifestyle. These chemicals can have profound effects on specific biochemical processes or simply promote the stress response and shift our state to become primed for inflammation. Below is a nonexhaustive list of some of the chemicals in our homes, food, and environments that we need to become aware of and try to avoid or eliminate as much as possible.

Food and Agriculture
- Pesticides, fungicides, and herbicides
- Hormones and antibiotics injected into farmed animals

Air and Water
- Runoff and release from industrial and agricultural sources
- Automobile fumes

- 2,4-D sprayed on the grass of golf courses, which runs off into the local water

Personal Care Products
- Aluminum in deodorant and antiperspirant
- Chemicals in makeup
- Benzenes in fragrances

Household and Consumer Products
- Plastics containing bisphenol A (BPA), bisphenol S (BPS), and other xenoestrogens
- Nonstick cookware lined with polytetrafluoroethylene (PTFE) and perfluorooctanoic acid (PFOA)
- Chemical cleaning supplies with highly reactive chemicals

Clothing and Fabric
- PFAS in sportswear, bedding, and tablecloths
- Flame-retardant chemicals in household fabrics

In addition to these biochemical stressors, we are also susceptible to other forms of stress that have not been considered by conventional health practitioners until very recently. These are not well understood or researched as yet but are stressors that need to be further evaluated and understood so as to help us limit the potential damaging effects.

Some of these include electromagnetic radiation such as Bluetooth and Wi-Fi networks, microwave ovens, cell phones, and cell phone networks. Do your best to be safe and avoid these not-yet fully understood sources of stress.

CHAPTER 6

ALLOSTATIC LOAD

What if there were a cumulative scoreboard of wear and tear that your body had to endure over time? This concept has been discussed and theorized in many books with valid points, including *The Body Keeps the Score* by Dr. Bessel van der Kolk and *When the Body Says No* by Dr. Gabor Maté. Let us briefly review the concept of allostatic load in this chapter.

HOMEOSTASIS

Homeostasis is the body's ability to maintain a stable internal environment from moment to moment by regulating various physiological processes. This concept is focused on keeping key physiological variables such as body temperature, blood glucose, hydration, and pH at optimal levels within a narrow range.

The mechanism by which homeostasis is achieved is through negative feedback loops. We have internal set points organized by central systems (mostly in the CNS), and any deviation from these set points are counteracted through physiological changes to bring the body back to equilibrium. The time frame of homeostasis is very short, concentrating on rapid moment-to-moment adjustments to return the body closer to the internal set points, resulting in stability.

A simple example of a homeostatic mechanism is when your body becomes warm, causing your internal body temperature to rise, and then your homeostatic mechanism of sweating will begin to attempt to cool you down and bring your body temperature back to the internal set point.

ALLOSTASIS

Allostasis is different from homeostasis in that it refers to the broader ability to achieve stability through adaptation to changing conditions over longer periods of time. This is a more nuanced and dynamic process of achieving stability in response to ongoing or anticipated challenges.

Allostatic mechanisms utilize activation of the nervous system, endocrine system, and immune system to prepare the body to respond effectively to current or upcoming stressors. Allostatic mechanisms are more complex, involving multiple systems coordinating to manage the physiologic response to present and future stressors. With this, allostasis operates over a longer time frame than homeostasis and must consider the cumulative effects of stressors and adaptations. The focus of allostasis is stability over time, even if that requires temporary deviations from the internal set points.

ALLOSTATIC LOAD

The allostatic load refers to the cumulative effect of stressors and adaptations over time that have resulted in "wear and tear" in the body. This is what is referred to in the books discussed at the beginning of this chapter and the amount of wear specifically has an effect on the capacity of the vagus nerve to handle the stress.

In an acute circumstance, the role of the VN is to relay information to remain in homeostasis, near the set point, but over time and accumulation of stressors, the VN can become less capable of handling stress as the "brakes wear down." The idea of the body keeping score is that the greater the allostatic load, the more stress the body has gone through, and the less capable it will be to handle future stressors. As such, the accumulation of stressors over time will actually result in an unwanted but necessary new set point or new normal.

This is exactly why we need to train our body to be capable of handling stress. The ability to recover from stressors is the role of the VN, and as we go through time, it is inevitable that we will experience stressors. The effect that these stressors have on us and our ability to rebound and come back as close to the initial set point is what determines the size of the allostatic load.

The best way to train our bodies to handle stress is through a concept called "hormesis." Hormesis is a biological phenomenon in which we expose ourselves purposefully to a small or moderate amount of stress (emotional, biochemical, or physical, being sure not to enter overload) and learn to actively bounce back to the set point, thus building our adaptive capacity, aka resilience. Learning to upgrade our vagus nerve to handle different forms of stress is the key to decreasing the effect of stress over time and lowering our allostatic load.

The reason why we assess all the different forms of stress and the effects that they have had on you throughout your life is to determine your relative allostatic load. We also want to know what tools you have used in the past and are using currently to build your adaptive capacity and help you to build your resilience so that you are well positioned to handle future stressors.

Within this area, we need to understand your mindset toward stress, which is a concept we will explore in the next chapter.

CHAPTER 7

PERCEPTION OF STRESS

Do you view stress as a bad thing? Are you personally able to experience a stressor as a positive challenge rather than an external obstacle that is keeping you down?

In her book *Mindset*, author Carol Dweck outlines the two basic forms of mindset that people tend to have, and how they perceive stressors or challenges. These mindsets are either "fixed" or "growth mindset."[6]

A fixed mindset has an inherent belief that intelligence or personal capacity is static and limited. The result of this fixed mindset is that challenges are looked at as impeding one's ability to live comfortably. People with a fixed mindset desire to look smart in front of others, and so they tend to focus only on things they already feel they can accomplish. As such, if there is something that they are not well versed on, they tend to avoid the challenge, give up easily, see efforts as fruitless, ignore constructive feedback, and often feel threatened by the success of others. People who live in this mindset are less willing to learn and grow, believing that the world is working against them.

On the other hand, a growth mindset is one that believes that intelligence is not static, but rather can be developed over time. These individuals have an inherent curiosity and desire to learn, which allows them to embrace challenges, persist through setbacks, and learn from criticism. They see effort as the path to mastery and find lessons and inspiration in the success of others around them.

Of all the factors involved in stress affecting the body, there is no question in my mind that individual perception of stress is by far the most important factor in determining the extent of breakdown that can occur.

People who believe that the challenge or stressor that they are facing is working against them (fixed mindset) tend to suffer more greatly from the effects of that stress than those who believe that the stressor is a challenge that they can overcome and learn from.

I have consulted with thousands of people in my practice, and I can say with near 100 percent confidence that this factor is the greatest determinant of how well a client will do in my program and if they will have long-term success. What you believe you are capable of is the single most important factor in being able to step up and face or succumb to the challenge.

Here are a few important questions to truly ask yourself and answer honestly as you begin your journey to upgraded health:

◆ Do I view my health as holding me back or as a challenge to overcome or learn from?
◆ Am I capable of and willing to step up to the challenge?
◆ Am I willing to let go of prior beliefs in the face of new information?

- Am I willing to use the new information I gain to make real changes in my life and habits?
- Am I willing to invest time, effort, and resources in creating the life I want to live?

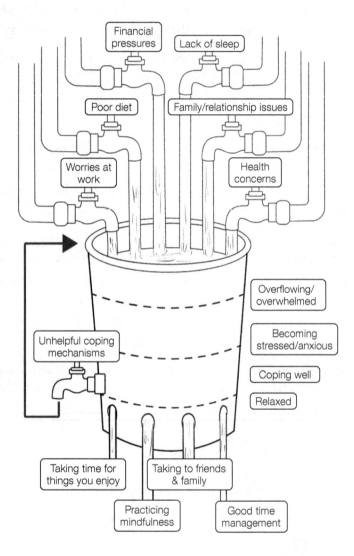

CASE STUDY: DIANE

Diane, a 57-year-old female former world-class figure skater, presented to my office in 2020 with a history of falls on the ice, causing concussions and being accompanied by migraine headaches. She was suffering from a host of symptoms for which she was seeing various specialists. Her symptoms included poor cognition and memory issues, mild depressed mood, bloating, occasional constipation, joint pain, and low energy. She had previously been diagnosed with hypothyroidism (Hashimoto's thyroiditis) and Raynaud's phenomenon, and had entered menopause about three years before coming to see me.

I took a thorough history and timeline of her health issues, which included secondhand smoke exposure in her childhood home, the use of mercury amalgam fillings for dental cavities as a child, chronic over-exercising in her teens and twenties associated with her figure skating career, and body image issues for which she had periods of eating disorders—both anorexia and bulimia: major stressors to the digestive tract and signaling in the VN. Diane also had three pregnancies and had given birth to four children (one set of twins); however, she had experienced a psychological trauma, having lost one of her children in 1993.

My clinical examination using functional lab testing revealed poor carbohydrate metabolism, poor detoxification capacity, and high bacterial toxin levels resulting from a leaky gut. Stool testing showed elevated levels of *Helicobacter pylori* bacteria in her stomach and the high levels of four different dysbiotic bacteria in her intestinal tract. She also had a very high intestinal inflammation finding called "calprotectin."

Diane experienced a significant number of stressors from many different sources—physical stress from multiple falls on the ice; biochemical stress from microbiome dysbiosis in her gut, amalgam fillings, and secondhand smoke exposure; psychological stress from her challenges with body image resulting in eating disorders, and quite significantly from the loss of her child. Many different stressors in each of the buckets pushed on the accelerator (sympathetic nervous system) and eventually caused the breakdown of the brakes (parasympathetic nervous system).

In Diane's case, we used nutritional therapy, cutting out some common inflammatory triggers; targeted probiotic therapy; supplements to support detoxification; and vagus nerve exercises with reasonably positive results in the first four weeks. She then began using a vagus nerve stimulator as well as herbal antibacterial therapy and had a very positive change in her health.

She revealed to me that approximately six weeks into our care program, it was as though "the light switch had turned back on," and she was feeling major improvements in her mood, sleep, and energy. Her joint pain had reduced quite significantly such that she was able to exercise again, which was very helpful for her mood. The game changer in her case was vagus nerve stimulation, which seemed to help shift her body into a state of recovery, allowing her to feel more capable and able to take on greater challenges.

Diane has continued to show improvement in her health and shared with me that it is like her brain has begun working again. She practices mindfulness daily, sees a traditional Chinese medicine practitioner weekly, and is following a ketogenic diet with intermittent fasting five days per week.

UNDERSTANDING AND MEASURING VAGUS NERVE FUNCTION

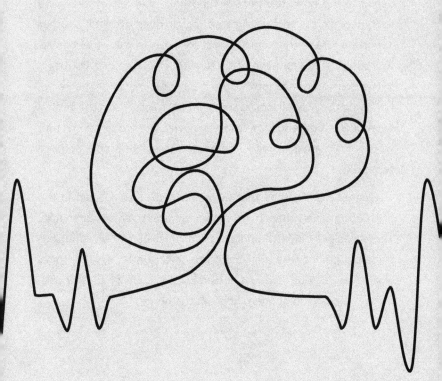

CHAPTER 8

PERIPHERAL VAGUS NERVE ANATOMY

The vagus nerve as we see it in the body is a peripheral nerve that begins in the brain stem and extends into the neck, thorax, and abdomen. This is technically true, but it does overlook another important area—the signals that are relayed into the central nervous system from the brain stem nuclei. First, we will begin in the brain stem and look at the peripheral course of the nerve. Following this, we will look at the neuronal tracts within the central nervous system, and how the vagus nerve circuits connect to various brain areas to modulate neurotransmitter production and release.

The peripheral neurons that form the vagus nerve begin in the brain stem, then branch from four different regions or nuclei. These nuclei include the dorsal motor nucleus of vagus, nucleus tractus solitarius (aka nucleus of the solitary tract—NTS), spinal trigeminal nucleus, and nucleus ambiguus. Each of these nuclei control specific component fibers of the nerve.

Sensory neurons bring signals from the skin that the vagus nerve innervates to the spinal trigeminal nucleus. This includes a specific section of skin of the ear via the tragus nerve.

Signals from the internal organs of the body are relayed via the NTS to be processed and then moved up into the brain for further processing. These signals are the parasympathetic afferent signals from the stomach, intestinal tract, lungs, heart, liver, gallbladder, pancreas, and spleen. Approximately 80 percent of the fibers in the vagus nerve perform this particular action, meaning that 80 percent of the information on the VN are functional status updates coming from the organs up to the central nervous system.

We are also able to send direct signals to these organs through the vagus, using parasympathetic efferent fibers, which originate in the dorsal motor nucleus. These signals help to calm and regulate the function of the heart and lungs and increase the action of the gut and other visceral organs listed above.

The final nucleus that contributes fibers to the vagus is the nucleus ambiguus. This nucleus sends out neurons that have a motor function, specifically working to control the majority of muscles present in the throat and upper airway. These muscles are responsible for keeping the airway open and producing sound using the vocal cords, thus creating your voice.

The right and left vagus are the only nerves in the body with four different functions and four distinct nuclei that relay different signals in both afferent and efferent directions.

Most other nerves in the body carry simple sensory information from the skin and/or motor signals for movement to the muscles.

This simple fact shows just how important this nerve is to the optimal function of the body.

Now, let's follow the path of the nerves from the brain stem, coursing downward into the neck, thorax (chest area), and the abdomen (belly area).

INTO THE NECK

From the brain stem region known as the "medulla oblongata," fibers of the left and right vagus nerves extend into the cranial cavity (essentially the inside of the skull) and converge to form the vagus nerve. The nerve then passes out of the skull through an opening called the "jugular foramen." This opening is a large space for the nerve and other blood vessels to pass through from the neck to enter the skull. Once the nerve exits the skull, it enters the subcranial area of the neck just behind the ear and is located between the internal jugular vein and internal carotid artery. These blood vessels are the direct contributors of blood to and from the brain and are critical in keeping us alive.

Immediately after the vagus passes through the jugular foramen, the nerve thickens to form the superior ganglion (or jugular ganglion).

A ganglion is a thickening of a nerve that is formed by a collection of sensory neuron cell bodies, located in very close proximity to one another. The cell bodies of the sensory nerves congregate in this ganglion, then re-form into the thinner nerve section, which gives rise to the first branch of the vagus nerve—the auricular branch.

The auricular branch then passes back into the skull through another opening called the "canaliculus" and toward the ear through yet another hole of the skull called the "tympanomastoid fissure." The nerve then extends toward the skin of the ear on each side of the body respectively. This branch senses touch, temperature, and wetness on the skin of the external canal, tragus, and auricle.

This branch of vagus is the main target for activation treatment of VN dysfunction using auricular acupuncture (acupuncture points in the ear), which we will discuss in later chapters.

As the nerve begins passing downward (or "inferiorly" in anatomist language) from the superior ganglion, the VN thickens once again to form the inferior ganglion (also known as the "nodose ganglion"). This ganglion houses the cell bodies of the neurons that are involved in bringing information from the internal organs. The nerve then thins out again and immediately enters a passageway created by a thickening of connective tissue called the "carotid sheath." Along with the internal carotid artery and internal jugular vein, these three structures are given extra soft-tissue protection as they pass down through the neck.

The carotid sheath is a dense band of fibrous connective tissue that contains the internal carotid artery, internal jugular vein, and the vagus nerve. This structure is imperative to our optimal function as it contains the two blood vessels tasked with bringing blood flow to and from the brain, along with the vagus nerve. Damage to this structure would result in significant challenges in the regulation of the body and dysfunction of the central nervous system as well as the relay of important signals of inflammatory control via the vagus nerve.

Within the carotid sheath, the vagus nerve gives off its next two branches, the pharyngeal and the superior laryngeal branches.

The pharyngeal branch has neurons from the vagus but also carries some contributing neurons from the ninth and eleventh cranial nerves (glossopharyngeal and accessory nerves). Once these neurons converge, they will pass toward the midline of the body until they reach the upper part of the throat, called the "pharynx." In the pharynx, the neurons of the VN relay motor signals to multiple muscles, which are involved in the swallowing reflex as well as managing the opening and closing of the upper airway and maintaining the gag reflex.

As the vagus nerve continues to descend along the sides of the neck within the carotid sheath, it gives rise to the third branch of the VN, known as the "superior laryngeal nerve." This nerve branches from the VN immediately after the pharyngeal nerve and supplies motor signaling to the muscles of the larynx above the vocal cords, specifically the muscles that control the pitch of your voice.

As the nerve courses down through the carotid sheath, it gives rise to the cervical cardiac branches of the VN, which are two of the three branches of this nerve to course toward and innervate the heart. The third branch, the thoracic cardiac branch, arises soon after leaving the carotid sheath—in the chest or thorax area. These branches intermingle with nerves of the sympathetic nervous system and form the cardiac plexus. A plexus is a collection of intermingling nerve fibers of different branches and different origin nerves that course toward a specific location. We have two cardiac plexi (plural of plexus), one in front of the aorta called the "superficial cardiac plexus" and one behind the arch of the aorta (in front of the trachea and bronchi of the lungs), called the "deep cardiac plexus."

In the case of these cardiac plexi, sympathetic and parasympathetic fibers come together and intermingle to form branches and extend toward specific areas of the heart. Some fibers extend toward the sinoatrial (SA) node of the heart, while others will extend toward the atrioventricular (AV) node. We will discuss the function of these nerves on the heart in the next chapter. For now, the most important thing to remember is that these fibers signal to control the rate of electrical activity that pumps your heart.

INTO THE THORAX (CHEST)

After the nerve exits the bottom of the sheath, it then continues to course downward into the thorax, behind the first and second ribs and in front of the larger blood vessels that extend from the heart.

The left VN passes in front of (anterior to) the arch of the aorta (the primary blood vessel carrying blood from the heart to the rest of the body) and then sends off its fourth branch—the recurrent laryngeal nerve.

Meanwhile, on the opposite side of the body, the right VN follows a similar path; however, it passes in front of the right subclavian artery (rather than the aorta) and then sends off its fourth branch, the right-side recurrent laryngeal nerve.

Both recurrent laryngeal nerves follow a similar path on opposite sides of the body. These are the only branches of the nerve that actually turn and course upward toward the neck again. They carry motor signals from the brain stem to each of the larynx muscles located below the vocal cords. These muscles function to activate the laryngeal muscles, creating tension in the vocal cords. This allows us to have pitch and tone in our voice. A monotone voice, or the inability to actively switch between high and low pitch while speaking, are an important and nuanced sign of VN dysfunction.

Also at the level of the aorta, each one of the vagus nerves sends off branches to the next pair of organs, the lungs. The left VN sends a pulmonary branch to the anterior pulmonary plexus, and the right VN sends a pulmonary branch to the posterior pulmonary plexus. These nerve branches mix with sympathetic neurons, reorganize, then travel to each side to innervate the lungs. These branches go to the bronchi and larger branches of the lungs to open and close them according to the need of the body based on each situation.

The thymus is one organ in the thorax that the vagus nerve innervates, which is imperative for optimal immune function but is overlooked due to its size in adulthood (see below). It is located in the mediastinum, essentially the chest area, in front of the heart but behind the sternum or chest bone. A branch of the VN courses to this organ to send immune regulatory signals to and from the thymus.

The thymus forms early in our development and is the major source of training for and growth of our white blood cells. The reason this organ is so easily forgotten is that, over time, it begins to shrink and be replaced with fat tissue. This process begins during puberty and can continue until the age of 40 to 50. I like to think of the thymus as a school for new immune cells, and as the school gets old and deteriorates, the training that the white blood cells go through decreases in quality.

INTO THE ABDOMEN

The final region that the VN innervates contains the organs of the abdomen. These are the primary digestive organs as well as those controlling the immune system and ensuring that the blood reaching the rest of our cells does not contain toxins that can negatively affect cell health.

The first of these branches goes to the stomach. When our body is in the parasympathetic rest-and-digest state (rather than the fight-or-flight, high-stress, or sympathetic states), the fibers of the VN work to stimulate stomach muscles to function. They send signals to the parietal cells to produce and secrete hydrochloric acid (HCl), the chief cells to produce and secrete pepsin and gastrin, and they send signals to the smooth muscle cells of the stomach to physically churn and push the food in our stomach into the next section of the digestive tract—the small intestine.

If the VN is damaged and not sending these important signals to the cells of the stomach, it will lead to issues such as gastroparesis (paralysis of stomach muscles) and/or hypochlorhydria (aka low stomach acid)—the latter is a major root cause of many health conditions. Sufficiently low pH for activating enzymes and breaking down food is produced by a healthy amount of stomach acid and secretion in the stomach. The optimal range of pH in the stomach should be around 3.0, while anything above 5.0 will not be strong enough to activate the digestive enzymes of the stomach, including pepsin and gastrin.

Low stomach acid does not allow the pH of the stomach to drop enough, thus interfering with food breakdown. This higher pH in the stomach can also allow unwanted bacteria, viruses, and parasites to make their way into the intestines and wreak havoc on your digestive tract.

The second abdominal branches extend to the liver. Interestingly, these branches to and from the liver are strongly linked to the sensation of hunger and desire for certain types of nutrients. The food that we eat initially enters the stomach to be broken down. It then proceeds to the small intestine, where most of our macro-nutrients (fats, carbs, and amino acids from protein) are absorbed into the bloodstream. These nutrients then flow into the liver via the portal vein for filtration, processing, and sending signals back up to the brain.

From the liver, the VN relays information regarding blood sugar balance, intake of fats, and information regarding liver function. In this capacity, the vagus nerve can also relay information regarding the amount of bile necessary to help in the digestion of fats. The liver has many functions that require vagus input, including and certainly not limited to production of bile salts (which are then sent to the gallbladder for storage); balancing the blood sugar through production of glucose; managing hunger and satiety through the measurement of fat intake; and filtration of the portal vein, which brings all nutrients and toxins from the gut as well as phase one and phase two of detoxification processes for fat-soluble hormones, neurotransmitters, and toxins from the body. The liver is very important to our overall well-being, and the VN innervation is strongly associated with maintaining this balance.

Intimately connected to the liver is the gallbladder. Often over-looked by the medical system (similar to the appendix), the gallbladder is important for optimal function of our bodies. When bile is produced in the liver and created in excess, the liver sends those bile salts to the gallbladder for storage, preparing for the next meal. When this next meal occurs, the gallbladder pumps bile into the duodenum (first part of the small intestine) to help absorb dietary fats into the bloodstream.

The pumping action of the gallbladder is mediated by the VN. One of the hepatic branches of the VN sends signals to the gallbladder, activating the smooth muscle cells in its walls, to pump bile out and into the digestive tract. This happens in response to a meal and determining from the taste buds (sensory receptors on the tongue) that fat is part of that meal and needs to be digested once it reaches the small intestine.

Gallbladder dysfunction, which we note symptomatically as gall-stones or gallbladder attacks (due to the presence of stones), is a direct sign of vagus nerve dysfunction. It occurs most commonly due to a lack of pumping action of the gallbladder. When the gall-bladder cannot pump out the bile that is present (due to reduced vagus nerve signaling), the bile becomes concentrated and forms salt crystals, which grow over time. If a salt crystal becomes lodged in the bile duct, the gallbladder becomes distended and leads to a significant amount of abdominal pain, usually below the ribs on the right side (however, the location of this pain can vary significantly). Gallbladder removal surgery, known as "cholecystectomy," is one of the most common surgical procedures around the world.

The next branch of the VN is directed toward the pancreas. Your pancreas is one of the most important glands in your body, with both an exocrine and endocrine component. The endocrine pancreas produces and secretes insulin and glucagon directly into the bloodstream to balance glucose levels in the blood (blood sugar). The exocrine pancreas produces and secretes digestive enzymes through a duct, directly into the small intestine. The three most notable digestive enzymes produced by the pancreas are protease, which breaks down proteins into their component amino acids; lipase, which breaks down fats from their component triglycerides into free fatty acids and cholesterol; and amylase, which breaks down carbohydrates into simpler sugars.

Vagus innervation sends signals from the pancreas back to the brain stem, relaying information regarding exocrine and endocrine cell status as well as signals from the brain stem back to the organ, relaying signals regarding food intake and which enzymes are required for production and release into the bloodstream and digestive tract. Vagus innervation is essential for relaying this information—a lack of signaling will alter the release of digestive enzymes, reducing the effectiveness of the digestive process.

Once the VN courses past the stomach, it forms the celiac plexus, which is a network formed between lumbar sympathetic nerves as well as the parasympathetic fibers of the VN. This network then sends branches to the remaining organs in the abdomen.

Innervation of the spleen is very unique and very important in the context of the VN. The function of the spleen is to house, train, and prepare immune cells that flow through the bloodstream. The splenic nerve is a sympathetic nerve that extends from the celiac plexus directly to the spleen. When sympathetic signals are flowing to the spleen, they are actually telling the spleen to keep white blood cells on high alert for foreign invaders or internal stressors. This is an important function, because without these signals, the spleen will not keep the immune cells trained and ready for battle when they are necessary.

The VN signals to the spleen are a major piece to the cholinergic anti-inflammatory pathway, as there are many tissues that the VN does not directly innervate, such as muscles, bones, and skin. In order to send inflammatory control signals, the VN works in conjunction with the spleen to spread the message through the bloodstream. VN signals are relayed through the sympathetic nerve to specific T cells in the spleen, asking them to turn on and spread more ACh throughout the body. There is much more to discuss on this topic, and I will do so in Chapter 11 on the cholinergic anti-inflammatory pathway.

After the celiac plexus, the next branch of the VN travels to the small intestine, the step of the digestive tract following the stomach. Once food has been broken down by the chemical and physical churning in the stomach, it enters the small intestine. Here it undergoes further digestive processing by the pancreatic digestive enzymes and bile.

The function of the small intestine is to break down and absorb the vast majority of our macronutrients. These include fats, carbohydrates, and proteins (which are ideally broken down into their component amino acids). The bloodstream receives the macronutrients that have been accepted by the lining cells of the small intestine.

The bolus of food must be pushed along the winding and coursing length of the small intestine. For this to happen, smooth muscle cells that line the entire digestive tract are activated by vagus nerve signaling the extensive network of nerves lining the digestive tract called the "enteric nervous system" (also known as "the second brain"), which triggers movement of food through the digestive tract.

One important thing to remember is that we have an immensely important relationship with other cells that are living in our digestive tracts. The relationship that I am speaking of is the symbiotic relationship between our human cells and the bacteria that are living in our gut—our microbiome.

The vast majority of our bacterial allies live in our large intestine—the thicker, shorter area of our digestive tract. The reason for this is that although these bacteria produce many important vitamins, minerals, and biochemical precursors for us, they *are* bacteria and can also produce many toxins as well as gas. We require a system that is able to keep these bacteria in check as well as relay signals to our brain regarding the status of digestive tract and microbiome function.

The vagus nerve activates smooth muscle cells to push this food along the remainder of the tract, but it also is the major relay path for the microbiome to speak with the brain. The vagus nerve innervates approximately the first half of the large intestine—the ascending and transverse portions.

The final organ innervated by the vagus nerve is actually two organs, with one located on each side of the body—the kidneys. These organs have a few different functions that are crucial to our health. The first is to filter the blood of any excess water and uric acid, which contains water-soluble toxins to be released from the body. The kidneys filter out this fluid and form urine, which they then send down to the bladder. One of the major determinants of this control is blood pressure. The vagus nerve is a major controller of the function of the kidneys and thus has a major role in the management of blood pressure as well.

At the end of its course, the vagus nerve does not simply terminate. It forms a final plexus with the parasympathetic nerves that extend from the lower end of the spinal cord. These fibers of parasympathetic control innervate the second half of the large intestine called the "descending colon" or "sigmoid colon," as well as the bladder and sex organs.

CHAPTER 9

VAGALLY MODULATED CNS TRACTS

When we think of the vagus nerve as well as most other nerves, it is easy to envision projections from the brain, brain stem, and spinal cord that connect to all areas of the body in the periphery. What is often overlooked are the projections from these nerves entering the central nervous system (again, brain, brain stem, and spinal cord) and the relay pathways by which this information is brought to various CNS areas for processing. These internal relay pathways can become quite complicated and have a lot of overlap, but I will simplify and focus on the pathway relayed internally from the nucleus of the solitary tract, as it is the most relevant for the release of many neurotransmitters in the brain and central nervous system.

As we have discussed, approximately 80 percent of vagus nerve fibers are afferent, meaning that they send signals from the body to the brain stem at the region of the medulla oblongata. The nucleus of the solitary tract (NTS for short due to its Latin name, *nucleus tractus solitarius*) is the primary nucleus to receive these inputs. The NTS is the beginning point of the cholinergic system within the CNS, allowing for the production and release of the important neurotransmitter acetylcholine, which we will revisit soon.

As these signals enter the NTS, they are first relayed via a neuronal tract to a region in the brain stem called the "locus coeruleus" (LC), which is a major thoroughfare of information in the brain and central nervous system. The LC is tasked with secreting an important neurotransmitter called "norepinephrine," which is involved in wakefulness, attention, and focus. The LC produces norepinephrine in response to signals coming in from the NTS via afferent vagus nerve fibers.

LC projections relay norepinephrine higher into the brain to eight particular areas to increase the function of these regions. Let's go through each of these areas to understand the internal effects of an optimal functioning vagus relay system in the brain. These functions were wonderfully summarized in an article from Bari et al. in 2020.[7]

1. Dorsal Raphe Nucleus (DRN)

The DRN is the primary source of serotonin production in the CNS. Serotonin is known as the mood-regulation molecule. It is produced in this region from the amino acid tryptophan and is later converted to melatonin. LC signaling to the DRN will increase the production and release of serotonin, resulting in mood regulation, and will support the conversion of serotonin to melatonin in the pineal gland, which aids in circadian regulation and sleep. This region is very important in the regulation of mental health.

2. Thalamus

The thalamus is a region of the brain located centrally below the corpus callosum and is highly involved in sensory input processing, stress detection, and pain modulation. The LC projects to a specific region called the "paraventricular thalamus" (PVT), which is critical in cognitive arousal and wakefulness as well as triggering motivated behaviors by increasing dopamine production and release. This area is also involved in the process of initiating consciousness following anesthesia. Innervation to the PVT from the LC (via vagal inputs) is necessary for wakefulness, consciousness, and focused motivated behavior.

3. Hypothalamus

The connections between the LC and hypothalamus are quite extensive and would take hours to tease apart to fully understand. The hypothalamus is located just below the thalamus in the brain and regulates autonomic function, endocrine hormone release, and the sleep-wake cycle. Breakdown of the hypothalamus and LC are involved in Alzheimer's disease and other neurodegenerative conditions.

In a very simplified summary, the connections between the LC and hypothalamus result in the regulation of the circadian rhythm, regulating gut motility to turn on or off (which is signaled down via the vagus nerve), and the coordination of hormones released from the pituitary gland (which is heavily regulated by the hypothalamus).

Less than optimal VN signaling through the LC to the hypothalamus can result in fatigue and dysregulation of hormones, including the adrenal hormones such as cortisol. The nuanced role of the HPA (hypothalamic-pituitary-adrenal) axis seems to be regulated when vagus inputs are functioning optimally. A recent study from Penn State College of Medicine showed that vagotomized rats had dysregulation of the HPA axis, resulting in suboptimal responses to acute stressors. A regulated stress response is of the highest importance in maintaining homeostasis and building resilience.[8]

4. Amygdala and Hippocampus

Connections from the LC also extend to the amygdala and hippocampus, two brain regions involved in emotional memories and learning, emotional control, and feeding behavior.

The amygdala is involved in creating emotions and conditioning a fear response. This area becomes highly dysregulated in post-traumatic stress disorder (PTSD), as the fear response circuits strengthen and the ability to reduce or eliminate this fear response becomes more difficult.

Stimulation of the vagus nerve has been shown to enhance the ability to break down the circuits that are involved in triggering inappropriate responses to acute stressors due to the patient's chronic fear-based responses. Microglial cells are the main cells to manage the plasticity of these neuronal connections, and they require acetylcholine to keep them in a homeostatic housekeeping state. Without sufficient vagus nerve signaling, the ACh levels are insufficient to keep these cells operating in a housekeeping manner, and this will lead to the inability to regulate the circuits that manage the fear response.

Neurons in the hippocampus regulate the ability to learn and increase our control of memories. There are direct and indirect connections from the vagus nerve through the NTS and LC to the hippocampus, which are involved in bringing gut-based signals to the brain. Vagus nerve stimulation has been shown to improve memory, cognition, and the ability to learn, by regulating activity in the hippocampus through increased inflammatory control. It does this by releasing Ach and brain-derived neurotrophic factor (BDNF). Optimal vagus innervation to the hippocampus enhances our ability to learn and regulate our memories more effectively.

5. Cerebellum

The cerebellum has many different functions, but the best understood function is the normalization and smoothening of movements through movement coordination. Norepinephrine (NE) from the LC helps ensure that the cerebellum is actively working and able to coordinate movements and fine-tune our coordination.

6. Prefrontal and Sensory Cortices

The connection to the prefrontal cortex helps to drive a process called "executive function." This helps us to maintain attention, optimize cognition and higher order functioning, and to read and react to social situations with behavioral flexibility. The prefrontal cortex is the region of the brain that is associated with high-order cognitive functions including processing and reasoning that we as humans have, separating us from other primates and mammals.

Optimal function of the vagus nerve will help to allow these higher order functions to occur in a timely manner. When the signaling from vagus is insufficient, the effect is a lower threshold for inflammation to occur, as the microglial cells will be primed toward inflammatory processing, which will often manifest as slower cognitive processing speed and an inability to think as clearly as one would like.

The sensory cortex receives signals from the peripheral nerves of the body, and sends those signals to be processed by other areas of the brain. These relayed signals can be used to initiate movements or other responses. Vagal inputs are involved in ensuring that sensory processing occurs in an effective manner, and that they are appropriate to the situation triggering the sensation. Inappropriate responses can manifest as hypersensitivity to touch. The diagnosis of fibromyalgia can also be involved in inappropriate processing at the sensory cortex due to the presence of excess inflammatory signals.

7. Substantia Nigra and Ventral Tegmental Area

The neurons in the substantia nigra are the primary sources of dopamine production in the brain and CNS. Dopamine is our motivation-and-drive molecule that signals us to strive toward achieving something. Dopamine as a neurotransmitter is involved in addiction and obsessive behavior. Dysfunction of these regions has been shown to occur in Parkinson's disease.

NE signals to the substantia nigra and ventral tegmental area to stimulate the production of dopamine in these neurons, allowing us to create behaviors of motivation and drive toward a goal. Optimal levels of dopamine are necessary for us to be able to work toward achieving that goal, and these regions are reliant on the input of NE from the LC to activate this pathway.

8. Basal Forebrain (Nucleus Basalis of Meynert and Medial Septal Nucleus)

The nucleus basalis of Meynert (nbM) and medial septal nucleus are the CNS primary sources of acetylcholine. As we will learn throughout this book, acetylcholine is an absolute necessity when it comes to modulating inflammation and immune cell activity. This is not only true in the periphery of the body, but even more so in the brain and central nervous system.

The nbM is the primary source of ACh in the cerebrum, while the medial septal nucleus sends its ACh primarily to the midbrain, cerebellum, and brain stem. The function of the ACh release from these nuclei is to modulate the activity of the tissue-resident immune cells—microglia and astrocytes, among others. We will explore this concept in depth in Chapters 10 and 11. Modulation of these cells helps to reduce their drive toward inflammation and keeps us in a state of rest, digest, and recover. We are able to remain in a state of homeostasis and optimal function when we have a suitable amount of ACh signaling from the vagus nerve to the NTS, then up to the LC, and finally to the nbM. The effective signaling of ACh is the crux of the function of the VN.

As the vagus nerve sends 80 percent of its signals up to the CNS via afferent fibers, the optimal function of the VN is highly correlated to optimal brain function, balanced mood, coordinated movements, and inflammatory control. The importance of uncompromised VN signaling to the brain cannot be overstated—especially when it comes to challenges of mental health, traumatic brain injury, neurodegenerative conditions, and recovery from highly stressful events.

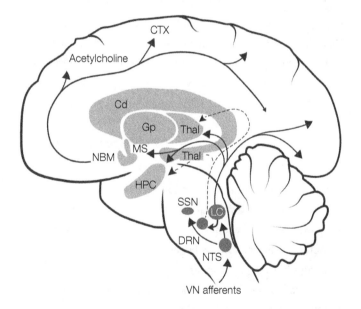

Cd - Caudate nucleus
CTX - Cerebral cortex
DRN - Dorsal raphe nucleus
Gp - Globus pallidus
HPC - Hippocampal formation

LC - Locus coeruleus
NBM - Nucleus basalis of Meynert
NTS - Nucleus tractus solitarius
MS - Medial septal nuclei
SSN - Superior salivatory nucleus
Thal - Thalamus

Of all the connections into the CNS that the vagus nerve has, I would note that the connection to LC and nbM are the most important for regulation of inflammation and optimal cognitive function. LC produces norepinephrine, creating focus and activation in many nuclei, while nbM is highly necessary for regulating the immune cells of the CNS—namely the microglia and astrocytes: cells that have been overlooked in terms of their importance to optimal brain function.

CASE STUDY: VLAD

Eighteen years ago, Vlad began experiencing some odd neurological symptoms. He began to lose his sense of smell, noticed that his voice was becoming weaker, and he started having a tremor in his right hand. Over time, he also noticed difficulty swallowing, experiencing a few mini-choking episodes, including one major episode just a few years before coming to see me. Countless appointments and tests over the next few years finally gave him an answer, as he was diagnosed with Parkinson's disease by his neurologist.

Vlad's wife, Renee, was curious to determine why this issue had occurred, since he didn't have any family history or apparent increased risk, including never suffering a concussion or detectable brain injury. She began to research and eventually became a holistic practitioner and nutritionist to see if she could help him identify the root cause of his deteriorating health.

When Vlad had his first call with me, he shared that he had tried many nutritional strategies that had helped his digestion, but he was feeling quite depressed and had a low mood most of the time. He had previously worked as a freelance film and video producer and director, but due to his diagnosis, neuro-logical challenges, and low energy, he had retired though still had a passion to create. He also truly wanted to support his family as best he could, but since he wasn't working, he was unable to contribute financially. He and Renee had read my first book and were interested in learning more about improving VN function, as it seemed linked to some of the neurological and health optimization findings.

Vlad had three goals he wanted to achieve: more energy, less tremor, and less body stiffness. He also wanted to become more organized and improve his depression and mental health. Vlad loves to play pickleball and does so regularly, but his energy following a match is always quite low.

We had a breakthrough in helping Vlad and his wife determine a major trigger to the health challenges and his diagnosis. Approximately two years prior to the onset of his initial symp-toms, Vlad and Renee's son had been in a major auto accident in which he was hit by a car and diagnosed with a severe traumatic brain injury (level 8 on the Glasgow Coma Scale, for the clinicians out there). The incident itself was psychologically very difficult for their family, and according to Renee, during the next year of rehabilitation, Vlad was the glue that held the family together.

This experience of needing to give of yourself and sacrifice your own needs to take care of others can be a major stressor, and that seems to have been the inciting stressor or triggering event that began the breakdown of Vlad's immune system and microglia in his brain. This was likely the event that triggered Vlad's diagnosis of Parkinson's disease.

After one week of using the recommended vagus nerve stim-ulation device along with other nutritional and supplemental therapies, Vlad messaged me saying he needed to talk. We immediately got on the phone and he shared some amazing news. He said that when he woke up that morning, he could smell Renee cooking bacon downstairs. This was the first time in nearly 18 years that he smelled something so profoundly since losing most of his sense of smell.

By stimulating Vlad's VN, we were able to send anti-inflammatory signals through the afferent pathways to the nucleus basalis of Meynert, activate the release of ACh, and send signals to the microglia to decrease their inflammatory activity. Signals would also be sent to the substantia nigra to support the production of dopamine, which is the area of the brain that is affected in Parkinson's disease.

CHAPTER 10

MACROPHAGES—THE TARGET CELLS OF THE VN

Since writing my previous book, I've often sat in contemplation regarding the exact mechanism by which such a simple system as the vagus nerve truly works to affect so many organs and cellular processes. This one question seemed to never be fully answered for me, as much of the research focused on different conditions that vagus nerve dysfunction was involved in.

In early 2022, I met JP Errico, the cofounder of electroCore Inc. This meeting was a turning point in allowing me to create a fuller and deeper understanding of the simplicity and complex nature of vagus nerve function and exactly how the VN could have such broad-reaching effects.

In my first dozen conversations with JP, we discussed everything regarding the vagus nerve and its target functions. This broadened my understanding and has increased my confidence as to the mechanism by which the VN breaks down, gets built back up, and the reasons why some people are able to overcome challenges quickly while others take much longer. Let's dig into the full understanding of the target cells of the vagus nerve: the marvelous macrophage! JP and I continue to have these amazing discussions on *The Health Upgrade Podcast*.

THE MISUNDERSTOOD IMMUNE SYSTEM

When most people think of the immune system, they think of the defense system of the body, protecting our organs from break-down caused by external threats to our survival or function. This is technically true; however, it is not the full picture.

There are two branches of the immune system—the innate and the adaptive.

The innate immune system is present from early in embryonic development and plays a vital role in shaping tissue formation, immune tolerance, and protection against pathogens. Although the fetus is in a relatively sterile environment, interactions with maternal cells and potential microbial exposures necessitate an active innate immune response. The innate immune cells, including macrophages, natural killer (NK) cells, dendritic cells, and neutro-phils contribute to various processes that we will dig into soon.

The adaptive immune system is a more specialized and sophisticated defense mechanism that develops during childhood and provides a tailored response to specific pathogens. It takes longer to activate but offers long-term immunity and memory. Upon encounter-ing a specific pathogen, the adaptive immune system generates memory cells that "remember" the pathogen. In subsequent encounters, the adaptive immune system mounts a faster and stronger response, providing long-term protection. The adaptive immune response involves specialized cells called "B lymphocytes"

(B cells) and "T lymphocytes" (T cells). B cells produce antibodies that target specific antigens, while T cells directly attack infected cells or coordinate immune responses.

While all immune cells will respond to signals from the vagus nerve, the macrophage component of the innate immune system is of utmost importance, as these cells are the housekeepers and maintenance staff of our tissues and organs.

WHAT IS SO SPECIAL ABOUT THE MACROPHAGE?

Upon conception, the process of cellular replication begins quite rapidly to form a human embryo. During this process, each of the pluripotent stem cells (cells with many potential differentiation pathways) begin to differentiate into specific cell types. Before these cells differentiate and specialize in becoming functional cells of each organ or system, they need a guide or manager to ensure that the differentiation process is working effectively, so that the right cells go to the correct areas and that the correct signals are released to promote cellular differentiation. Macrophages are the innate immune cell type that are highly involved in guiding these processes.

During human embryonic development, macrophages originate from two primary sources: the yolk sac and the fetal liver. During the early stages of development, macrophages derived from the yolk sac are the first wave of macrophages to appear in the developing embryo. They arise between days 16 and 19 after fertilization and play a crucial role in tissue remodeling, angiogenesis (the formation of blood vessels), and hematopoiesis (the formation of blood cells).

As embryonic development progresses, macrophages from the yolk sac are gradually replaced by macrophages derived from the fetal liver around week four or five of gestation. They replace the yolk-sac-derived macrophages and contribute to tissue remodeling, immune modulation, and clearance of apoptotic cells. During mid to late embryonic development, macrophages from the fetal liver migrate and infiltrate various tissues, where they undergo tissue-specific differentiation and form the resident macrophages of each organ in which they reside.

Differentiation of macrophages in specific tissues occurs as they respond to local signals and cues. These macrophage populations acquire unique phenotypes and functions adapted to their respective organ and tissue environments. Developmental macrophages are the main cells to manage the cellular differentiation of stem cells into different groupings that will eventually work together as organs.

These macrophages do not simply manage the development of the organs and then pack up and leave. They actually take up residence in each of these organs as we grow, and they remain there throughout our lives. Due to their differentiation at each organ, they have been given many different names, however they all have the same general functionality within each of these organs. These cells are known as tissue-resident macrophages. Here is a list of all the tissue-resident macrophages within the body.

TISSUE-RESIDENT MACROPHAGES IN THE BODY*

Organ	Tissue-Resident Macrophage	Dysfunction/ Involvement
Central nervous system	Microglia	Neurodegenerative disease
Lungs	Alveolar macrophages	Asthma, respiratory infections

TISSUE-RESIDENT MACROPHAGES IN THE BODY*

Organ	Tissue-Resident Macrophage	Dysfunction/ Involvement
Liver	Kupffer cells and motile macrophages	Non-alcoholic fatty liver disease (NAFLD), Non-alcoholic steatohepatitis (NASH)
Skin	Langerhans cells	Psoriasis, eczema, rashes
Kidney	Kidney-resident macrophages and glomerular mesangial cells	Polycystic kidney disease, kidney fibrosis
Heart	Resident cardiac macrophages	Myocarditis
Blood vessels	Vascular macrophages	Cardiovascular disease
Stomach	Gut intestinal macrophages	Hypochlorhydria
Small intestine	Intestinal macrophages	Intestinal hyperpermeability
Large intestine	Intestinal macrophages	Inflammatory bowel disease
Skeletal muscle	Muscularis macrophages	Cachexia, muscle breakdown
Bone	Osteoclasts	Osteoporosis
Connective tissue	Histiocytes	Ehlers-Danlos syndrome (EDS)
Ovaries	Ovarian macrophages	Polycystic ovarian syndrome (PCOS)
Uterus	Uterine macrophages	Endometriosis
Testes	Testicular macrophages	Male infertility
Spleen	Red pulp macrophages and white pulp macrophages	
Adrenal glands	Adrenal macrophages	HPA axis dysfunction
Pancreas	Pancreatic islet macrophages	Type 1 diabetes

TISSUE-RESIDENT MACROPHAGES IN THE BODY*

Organ	Tissue-Resident Macrophage	Dysfunction/ Involvement
Bloodstream	Circulating monocytes	Blood cancers
Peritoneum	Peritoneal macrophages	
Adipose tissue	Adipose-associated Macrophages	Obesity-related inflammation

* Source: M. K. Lee et al., "The Role of Macrophage Populations in Skeletal Muscle Insulin Sensitivity: Current Understanding and Implications." *International Journal of Molecular Science* 24, no. 11467 (2023), https://doi.org/10.3390/ijms241411467.

Tissue-resident macrophages play some crucial roles within each of the organs they reside once we have completed the full development stage. I consider these parallel to the roles of the repair, maintenance, housekeeping, and security teams that maintain a building.

Tissue maintenance and repair: Tissue-resident macrophages contribute to tissue maintenance and repair processes. They remove cellular debris, promote tissue remodeling, and aid in wound healing by producing growth factors and extracellular matrix components.

Immune surveillance: Tissue-resident macrophages serve as sentinels, constantly monitoring the local microenvironment for potential threats. They detect and engulf pathogens, preventing their spread within tissues. Tissue-resident macrophages play a role in antigen presentation, which can activate the adaptive immune response when necessary.

Immunological memory: Tissue-resident macrophages can develop immunological memory. They retain information about previous encounters with pathogens, allowing for faster and more effective responses upon reinfection.

Modulation of inflammation: Tissue-resident macrophages regulate inflammatory responses. They can initiate or dampen inflammation depending on the context, preventing excessive inflammation while maintaining the ability to respond to infections or injuries. This is particularly important when it comes to the development of chronic disease states, as uncontrolled inflammation is the pathway to many of these lifestyle-based conditions.

Tissue-specific functions: Different organs and tissues have specialized functions, and tissue-resident macrophages contribute to these functions. They communicate and interact with all of the other cell types within their resident organ and microenvironment. They communicate with neighboring cells, such as fibroblasts, endothelial cells, and immune cells, through the release of cytokines, growth factors, and other signaling molecules.

In the gut, intestinal macrophages perform all of the stated above tasks, while also signaling to the epithelial lining cells, to produce zonulin and occludin, the molecules necessary for maintaining gut barrier integrity. In the central nervous system, microglia perform the task of neuronal synaptic pruning to manage and support neuroplasticity. Tissue-resident macrophages are the support staff that ensure each organ and tissue works effectively.

Macrophages all express a very particular receptor on their cellular surface—the a7 nicotinic acetylcholine receptor (a7 nAChR), which is the crux of the signaling mechanism by which the vagus nerve manages the function and state of these macrophages.

The role of the autonomic nervous system and, in particular, the vagus nerve is in managing the functional state of these tissue-resident macrophages. When the vagus nerve is working well and acetylcholine is being released, the a7 nAChR becomes activated. When this happens, there are three specific pathways that become activated and turn on the cholinergic anti-inflammatory pathway. We will go over this functionality very soon.

For now, note that the signaling of acetylcholine is necessary to shift the state of these macrophages into anti-inflammatory state, and a lack of ACh will result in priming of these cells toward a hyperinflammatory state.

The role of tissue-resident macrophages is as the security and maintenance teams for each organ in which they reside. There are some circumstances in which this functionality is insufficient, in which case, they require the services of specialized support cells that also happen to be immune cells. Recruiting of these additional support cells is akin to a security team calling for support from the police, firefighters, and emergency medical staff. Circulating monocytes are macrophages that roam through the bloodstream and respond to calls for help just like firefighters do when we need their support.

CIRCULATING MONOCYTES

When the tissue-resident macrophages detect a threat or challenge that they are incapable of handling themselves, they will call out to the rest of the immune system for support. Both the innate and adaptive immune system are present and roaming in the bloodstream, ready to support when they are called upon. Tissue-resident macrophages will send signals called "cytokines" into the bloodstream and interstitial spaces, which essentially act as an emergency call to 911.

The signals will be picked up by the immune cells that are roaming, including monocytes, lymphocytes, eosinophils, basophils, and neutrophils.

Lymphocytes are adaptive immune cells and can be classified as B cells or T cells. They mount an antigen-specific attack on the threat to eliminate that threat almost like a police officer that is more discerning in its approach to determine the correct threat to neutralize.

Eosinophils, basophils, and neutrophils are granulocytes, derived from the same innate immune cells as macrophages and mono-cytes, but they produce and release specific granules of enzymes to attack and neutralize different threats. They are named based on the color they show when they have been stained during histo-logical examination. Eosinophils tend to attack invading bacteria and parasites such as worms and protozoa and tend to induce a histamine response. Basophils tend to react more toward allergens and environmental toxins. Neutrophils act against bacterial and fungal infections. We can consider granulocytes to be specialized firefighters working to neutralize specific threats.

Monocytes are the closest relative to macrophages, and they circulate in the bloodstream awaiting the call to support via inflam-matory cytokines. They become activated when they come in contact with these cytokines and will begin to enter the affected tissue to put out the proverbial fire.

Monocytes are not very discerning and do not take quite as much time to assess the situation. In the same way that firefighters will come in and shut down the threat as quickly as possible, monocytes will do exactly that within the affected tissue. This is an import-ant functionality to have and one that we need to ensure survival, however it is not the best when it comes to fixing any damage.

If you were to experience a fire in your house, you would want to call the firefighters to come in and extinguish the flames as quickly as possible to limit the extent of damage and eliminate the threat that triggered the fire also as quickly as possible. Once the threat has been neutralized, you would then ask the firefighters to leave and for the repair team to come do their best work to fix the damaged caused by the fire as well as the damage caused by the firefighters. In order the stop the blaze, the firefighters must use water and various tools to save important things and get to the source to shut it down. In doing so, they will inevitably cause damage to the property as well, something that monocytes also do when they enter tissues to eliminate the inflammatory trigger.

The job of the monocyte is to put out the fire, and the job of some of the tissue-resident macrophages is to repair the damage that has been done. The specific signal required to turn off the monocytes and turn on the tissue-resident macrophages is an all-clear signal from the autonomic nervous system and the vagus nerve, in the form of acetylcholine. The system that manages this signaling is called the "cholinergic anti-inflammatory pathway."

NONINFLAMMATORY FIX MACROPHAGES

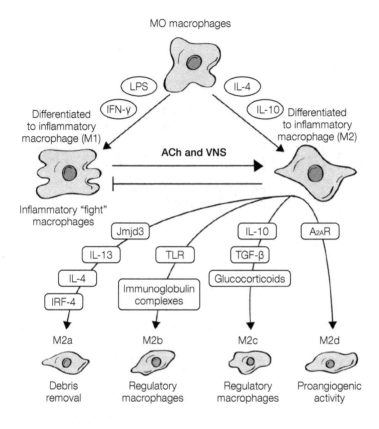

MO macrophages

LPS IFN-γ

Differentiated to inflammatory macrophage (M1)

IL-4 IL-10

Differentiated to inflammatory macrophage (M2)

ACh and VNS

Inflammatory "fight" macrophages

Jmjd3

IL-13

IL-4

IRF-4

M2a

Debris removal

TLR

Immunoglobulin complexes

M2b

Regulatory macrophages

IL-10

TGF-β

Glucocorticoids

M2c

Regulatory macrophages

A2AR

M2d

Proangiogenic activity

CHAPTER 11

THE CHOLINERGIC ANTI-INFLAMMATORY PATHWAY

The cholinergic anti-inflammatory pathway (CAIP) is a system that has been discovered over the past two decades, initially by Dr. Kevin Tracey and his research team at the Feinstein Institutes for Medical Research in Manhasset, New York.

This pathway is the functional relay circuit between the nervous system and the immune system—the neuroimmune system, if you would. At one end of the circuit, we have the central nervous system, which is made up of the brain, brain stem, and autonomic nervous system (parasympathetic and sympathetic branches). On the other side of the circuit, we have the tissue-resident macrophages and innate immune system.

The tissue-resident macrophages present in all tissues throughout the body are working as sentinels, constantly monitoring the functionality and assessing threats to the function of the cells. Anything that pushes the function out of an optimal state and threatens homeostasis must be identified and assessed in a timely manner. Threats to the optimal function of cells include all stressors we discussed in the first section of this book: psychological stressors, physical stressors, biochemical stressors, and daily stressors all potentially contribute to pushing tissues out of optimal function.

These stressors activate immune cell function in the form of inflammatory cytokines — signaling molecules used to draw attention to the affected tissues. This will locally trigger the activation of circulating immune cells such as monocytes, lymphocytes, and granulocytes depending on the specific cytokines being expressed.

The inflammatory cytokine signals will then also be sent through the afferent neurons of the vagus nerve up to the brain stem, namely the nucleus of the solitary tract. This information is constantly being assessed by autonomic and higher brain centers, sending info up to various nuclei. When stressors are identified, our brain processes the information and determines next steps, sending efferent information through spinal nerves if the stressor requires physical movement, and through autonomic efferent nerves to all the organs to change the state of your body depending on which relay circuits are turned on — sympathetic or parasympathetic.

Efferent information sent via the sympathetic nervous system puts us in a fight/flight state, which is outside of the CAIP, as this activation contributes to further inflammatory cytokine release and activation of more immune cell function. There are instances where this is necessary, but in a longer-term situation, this is highly inflammatory and the cause of chronic disease. Chronic sympathetic states are the driving force behind uncontrolled inflammation in the body.

When the CAIP is working correctly, the efferent signals are sent through the vagus nerve to have positive peripheral effects on the body, specifically to control inflammation. The effector molecule for this system is unsurprisingly, acetylcholine (hence "cholinergic"). The VN releases ACh directly to the tissue-resident macrophages in the organs that the VN directly innervates. There are, however, many tissues that are not directly innervated by the VN. In order to get the ACh signal to those tissues, the VN has a relay system that is crucial for inflammatory control, via the spleen. It is odd though that the VN does not have a direct parasympathetic branch to the spleen.

The VN sends a branch to the celiac ganglion, an important collection of *sympathetic* neurons that are part of the sympathetic chain ganglia, running just anterior to the spine on both sides. The celiac ganglion is located at the spinal level of the twelfth thoracic and first lumbar vertebrae, (T12-L1), the junction between the thoracic and lumbar sections of the spine.

Sympathetic nerves from the celiac ganglion course via a direct branch to the spleen, which is called the "splenic nerve." There are no parasympathetic fibers on this nerve, but the VN can essentially override the signals on this nerve when there is a need to control inflammation.

Sympathetic signals to the spleen via splenic nerve help to ensure that the spleen is on high alert and essentially training the immune cells to be ready to attack at a moment's notice. These signals are necessary but also need to be kept in check so as not to attack innocent cells that may resemble threats. To regulate those, the VN sends signals and releases acetylcholine at the celiac ganglion. ACh release at the celiac ganglion triggers splenic nerve activation and the release of norepinephrine (NE) in the spleen. NE release at the spleen is necessary to activate a very special kind of receptor cell found only at the junction of the splenic nerve and the spleen called the "ChAT cell."

ChAT cells are T lymphocytes, part of the adaptive immune system, that express an important receptor for this process, called the "b2-adrenergic receptor" (b2AR). When the b2AR is activated in these ChAT cells, they become signaling cells that produce and release acetylcholine into the spleen and throughout the rest of the body via the bloodstream. ChAT cells work as the amplifier for the signals from the VN to reach all the tissues in the body, resulting in reduced inflammatory cytokine signaling.

HOW DOES ACETYLCHOLINE WORK TO CONTROL INFLAMMATION?

At the cellular level, there are three pathways that are activated by acetylcholine, which work to reduce inflammatory cytokine release and control inflammation overall.

ACh attaches to the a7n AChR (nicotinic ACh receptor) located on the cellular surface, which activates signaling pathways inside the cell. There are two signaling pathways that directly affect the nucleus and DNA transcription of inflammatory cytokines.

The first pathway affecting the DNA transcription of inflammatory cytokines is the cAMP-c-fos pathway, which downregulates the transcription of NF-kB, which decreases the release of inflammatory cytokines TNFa, interleukin-1 (IL-1), and interleukin-6 (IL-6).[9]

The second pathway is the JAK2/STAT3 pathway, which downregulates the transcription of genes producing many different cytokines, many of which have been implicated in cancer treatments. The JAK2/STAT3 pathway is a major target for cancer therapies and is a specific target for inflammatory control via the CAIP.

The third pathway by which ACh creates an anti-inflammatory effect is, to me, the most significant and the most fascinating by far. This pathway still involves the a7 nAChR; however, this receptor is not located on the surface of the cell but rather inside the cell, on the surface of mitochondria, the energy production organelle within the cell.

This finding is quite new and very exciting to be able to understand the mechanism by which the VN affects cellular health and mitochondrial function.

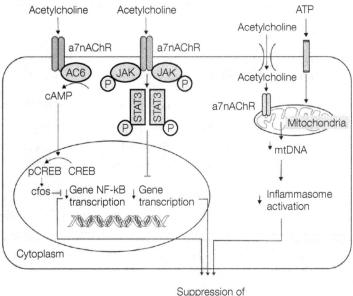

Suppression of
cytokine production

One of the main processes by which inflammation is activated is through a cellular mechanism called the "inflammasome." An inflammasome is a multiprotein complex that acts as a sensor of intracellular signals to trigger a cascade of inflammatory activation if the sensor becomes activated.

In the same way that our immune cells express cytokine receptors on their surfaces, allowing them to respond to extracellular inflammatory cytokines, the inflammasome works as a receptor within the cell to identify the presence of certain signals that indicate the cell is no longer working properly. It is a way to ensure the checks and balances of optimal function are ongoing. When a properly functioning inflammasome is activated, it triggers a cascade of cellular effects to release inflammatory cytokines extracellularly, essentially calling other immune cells to the area to eliminate a cell that is no longer working properly.

The most thoroughly studied inflammasome is the NLRP3 (NOD-like receptor protein 3); however, there are others: the ASC (apoptosis-associated speck-like protein containing a CARD), and caspase-1. For a short moment, we will focus on NLRP3.

NLRP3 is an intracellular receptor protein that responds to the presence of three major types of cellular dysfunction:

1. Ion Fluxes

Each of our cells is highly responsive to the presence of specific ions both inside and outside the cell. Ions form the basis of cellular charges (positive and negative) on either side of the cellular membrane, which allows for balance and optimal function. The ions that form this charge across the cell membrane include sodium ($Na+$), potassium ($K+$), calcium ($Ca2+$), and chloride ($Cl-$).

If there are any major changes to the presence of specific ions on either side of the cell membrane (due to dehydration, low electrolyte levels in the body, or excessive action of an ion channel), this will trigger activation of the NLRP3 inflammasome and lead to release of inflammatory cytokines into the extracellular space.

2. Lysosomal Damage

Lysosomes are sacs of enzymes that reside in certain cell types—mostly immune cells that use phagocytosis (aka cell eating) as their mechanism of action—macrophages being high on this list.

These sacs of enzymes can be dangerous to the cell that houses them, and as such they need to be kept in check. If these structures become damaged inside the cell, it can lead to various disease processes that can harm many other cells. As such, any detected damage to a lysosome will immediately trigger the inflammasome to enable cellular death or autophagy so as to limit damage to just the affected cell.

3. mtDNA Release or mtROS

Mitochondria function to turn carbs, fats, and proteins into ATP, meeting the energetic needs of the cell for optimal function. Mitochondria also contain their own DNA (known as mitochondrial DNA or mtDNA), which are provided solely by our mothers.

Damage to the mtDNA by reactive oxygen species or other toxic stressors will result in the mitochondria releasing their mtDNA into the cytoplasm of the cell. The NLRP3 inflammasome is highly sensitive to the presence of mtDNA in the cellular space, and as such it will trigger the full inflammasome cascade if damaged mtDNA is sensed by the NLRP3.

Since 2014, a number of studies have been released showing that mitochondria actually express their own a7 nAChR on their membranes. ACh can actually enter the cell directly when there is a surge of ATP present outside the cell, allowing the ACh to permeate the cell membrane and bind to the receptor on the mitochondrial membrane. When this mitochondrial version of the a7 nAChR is activated, it has been shown to significantly reduce the release of mtDNA, thus inhibiting the inflammasome and significantly lowering the presence of inflammatory cytokines.[10]

There are two circumstances that need to be fulfilled for this specific mechanism to become active. First, we need to have the presence of ACh outside the cell in reasonably high quantities — we can't be deficient in acetyl-CoA or choline, and we need to have an upgraded or effectively functioning vagus nerve. Secondly, we need a release of ATP from excitatory mechanisms taking place in the local tissue—this will occur during higher states of excitation and inflammation. This mechanism is the most fascinating as it may be involved in many chronic health conditions without a conventionally known cause or cure just yet.

Vagus nerve stimulation has been shown in recent studies to have a direct effect on lowering inflammasome activity. VNS is a therapy that is highly promising to help reduce inflammatory activity, and decreasing inflammasome activation is one of the most important mechanisms by which VNS can work to address chronic inflammatory conditions. We will dig deeper into VNS in Chapter 15.

CHAPTER 12

FUNCTIONS OF THE VAGUS NERVE—OVERVIEW

I spent the majority of my previous book, *Activate Your Vagus Nerve*, outlining the functions of the nerve—a topic I don't think we need to fully dig back into. Below is a short overview of VN functions that you should be aware of to begin understanding the next steps of how vagus nerve activation works to optimize health.

HEART RATE CONTROL

The most basic but important function of the VN in the body is regulation of the heart rate. Without any innervation to the heart, this unique organ has its own innate electrical rhythm to regulate its rate of beating. If there were no sympathetic or parasympathetic nerves connecting to the heart, it would beat at approximately 100 beats per minute (bpm). The role of the sympathetic innervation is to increase the heart rate in response to stress or challenge. The role of the parasympathetic innervation to the heart, via the vagus nerve, is to lower the heart rate.

The counterbalance between the sympathetic and parasympathetic innervation is what allows for variability in the timing between beats of the heart, a very important measure known as heart rate variability. This is a sign of resilience and autonomic nervous system balance.

As a basic overview, resting heart rate is a simple way to measure the number of heartbeats per minute and should generally be in the range of 50–65 bpm at rest. The lower the number (within this range), the greater the efficiency of blood flow with each beat of the heart, meaning that your heart literally doesn't have to work as hard to pump the required quantity of blood to the rest of the body. Highly effective cardio athletes can have even lower heart rates in the 40–50 bpm range, but in the general population, this number could be mildly indicative of a situation called "bradycardia" (literally meaning slow heart rate). The lowering of the heart rate to the optimal numbers of 50–65 bpm is mediated directly by the vagus nerve.

A resting rate of greater than 70 bpm becomes concerning, as it is a sign of sympathetic signals being stronger than parasympathetic signals. As a clinician, when I see this scenario, I immediately begin to look for hidden stressors in the life of my client, as there is clearly some burnout in the function of the parasympathetic signaling via the VN. When we exercise, move, or work and have elevated levels of the stress hormone cortisol, it actively accompanies an elevation in the heart rate as well. This is precisely why it is important to measure the resting vs. active heart rate and know that there is a distinction.

A chronically elevated heart rate is a direct sign of vagus nerve dysfunction.

A great way to assess the signaling capacity to the heart is to measure the difference in heart rate between the end of a workout or fitness test and one minute following the exercise—a measure known as "heart rate recovery." This measurement tool will be discussed further in Chapter 13, "Measuring Vagus Nerve Function."

MICROBIOME-GUT-BRAIN AXIS

The afferent pathway (body-to-brain direction) is the most prevalent pathway that information passes in the VN, and the greatest source of that information is from the gut and the microbiome. It is no coincidence that the largest percentage of immune cells by volume in the body is within the lining of the intestinal tract. We now know that the main signals on the VN are signaling to and from the immune cells, and thus this pathway is certainly not one to overlook.

There are approximately 80 to 100 trillion bacteria present in the intestinal tract of a human adult. For context, the human body has between 40 and 60 trillion human cells total, so it stands to reason that the population balance and signaling from the microbiome is of high concern and consequence to our well-being.

We previously mentioned that the microbiome contains both important symbiotic (beneficial) bacteria known as keystone bacteria and other opportunistic dysbiotic or even pathogenic bacteria, viruses, yeast, and parasites that are known to create inflammatory reactions when their quantities are not controlled.

Here are the names of some of the best-known keystone bacteria that we need to ensure good quantities of in our gut: *Lactobacillus* species, *Bifidobacterium* spp., *Enterococcus* spp., *Akkermansia muciniphila, Faecalibacterium prausnitzii, Roseburia* spp., *Rumino-coccus bromii, Methanobrevibacter smithii, Bacteroides* spp., and *Christensenella minuta.* Together, these species are known to break down complex carbohydrates, fiber, and resistant starches, providing us with short-chain fatty acids such as butyrate. They metabolize bile acids, support lipid metabolism, and metabolize tryptophan to support the production of serotonin, and this list is certainly not exhaustive when it comes to the symbiotic supports that these bacteria provide.

On the other hand, dysbiotic bacteria are a source of stressful by-products that can be damaging to the mucus barrier and epithelial lining, and a trigger for inflammatory reactions within the base layers of the gut. Some of the more common dysbiotic bacteria include *Helicobacter pylori, Streptococcus* spp., *Staphylococcus aureus, Morganella* spp., *Pseudomonas* spp., *Klebsiella* spp., *Prevotella* spp., and many others. The major toxin that these bacteria produce and cause issues with is called "lipopolysaccharide" (LPS for short), which is a known and well-researched toxin. We want to keep the LPS in the lumen of the gut and not allow it to breach the walls of the intestinal tract, as LPS is the main inflammatory trigger for the immune cells in the deeper layers. Continuous or long-term exposure to LPS is a major source of inflammation in those suffering from chronic disease.

There are also parasitic, viral, and fungal species that we need to be cognizant of, as they are major sources of digestive dysfunction and nutritional depletion. The presence of high levels of any of these dysbiotic bacteria, parasites, viruses, or fungi can severely diminish the capacity of our intestinal tract to keep out inflammatory triggers and absorb necessary nutrients from our food.

The functional status of these microbiome components is signaled up to the brain via the VN for assessment and coordination. If the VN is overburdened with other stressors and challenges to address, then it becomes less capable of sending this important info to the brain, and we are unable to respond to these triggers in a timely or effective manner.

DIGESTIVE SYSTEM

On the efferent side of the pathway, signals from the brain and the VN down to the gut initiate important action steps for the optimal function of the gut.

In the stomach, signals from the CNS stimulate the physical churning of food that has been eaten, as well as the release of stomach acid from the parietal cells in the lining of the stomach. This section is important as it is a critical step in the breakdown of our foods after we physically chew the food and provide saliva to help begin breaking the food down in the mouth and esophagus. Stomach acid (hydrochloric acid) is critical in the chemical break-down process of digestion.

A condition in which lower levels of hydrochloric acid is released is called "hypochlorhydria" and is much more common than most clinicians realize. Stomach acid is not only required for the chemical breakdown of food, but it also functions to sterilize and limit the amount of bacteria or other invaders that can enter the small intestine. Insufficient levels of stomach acid can result in a common challenge called "small intestinal bacterial overgrowth" (SIBO).

Another condition is called "gastroparesis"—in which the physical churning of the stomach is severely compromised due to a lack of VN signaling and reactivity within the muscular layers of the stomach itself. The physical motility of the digestive tract, including the stomach, is modulated both by a stretch response in the stomach and signals from the CNS via the VN to let the gut know that we are in a parasympathetic state that desires digestion to take place. Digestion is an energy-intensive process, and so it is important that we are in a state or situation that does not require the energy available to be used for a fight-or-flight response.

If we are chronically eating in a sympathetic state, or if there is damage or dysfunction to the VN, both conditions can be the result and cause major disruption to the correct functioning of the entire digestive tract.

Signals through the VN will also go to the exocrine part of the pancreas to stimulate the release of digestive enzymes, namely protease (to break down proteins), amylase (to break down carbohydrates), and lipase (which aids the breakdown of fats). These digestive enzymes are ideally released into the first part of the small intestine called the "duodenum," which begins the process of absorption of macronutrients into the body.

Low levels of VN signaling will often result in insufficient release of digestive enzymes, compromising the optimal breakdown and absorption of macronutrients from the small intestine. Pancreatic elastase is an important stool test marker to assess to determine if this is a challenge for you. Pancreatic insufficiency is also very common and should be supported through VN exercises and supportive upgrades.

In the intestines themselves, the VN signals support peristaltic motions of the intestines to move a bolus of food through the gut unidirectionally. In order to pass the bolus of food along the tube of the intestinal tract, signals are sent to the muscular layers within the walls of the gut lining to stimulate smooth muscle cells to contract and push the bolus in one direction. Suboptimal signaling results in a lack of motility in the gut and can cause the food to either be released too slowly or too quickly. This issue will not allow the optimal time required to digest and absorb the nutrients held in that food.

VN signals also go to the small intestine when we have not eaten any food and are in a fasting state, to trigger an important housekeeping function for the gut called the "migrating motor complex" (MMC). The MMC is stimulated by the optimal function of the VN along with hormones called "motilin" and "ghrelin" in a phased and coordinated cycle lasting approximately 113–230 minutes, depending on the person. The MMC functions to ensure the contents of the intestinal tract are kept optimal, not allowing bacteria to accumulate in the small intestine lumen and ensuring that we don't have a buildup of contents from the stomach making their way in.

If the MMC is not functioning optimally due to a lack of effective signaling through the VN or low levels of motilin or ghrelin hormone release, then the effect is a likely buildup of food and bacterial content in the small intestine that we previously discussed—SIBO. The root cause of SIBO comes down to a dysfunctional MMC due to lack of signaling through the VN.

The large intestine is mostly innervated by sacral and coccygeal parasympathetic nerves, but the signals are the same as those from the VN, ensuring optimal movement of foods and breakdown materials that need to be released from the body in a timely and efficient manner.

More than 2,000 years ago, Hippocrates stated that "All disease begins in the gut."[11] An optimal functioning digestive tract and microbiome-gut-brain axis are truly paramount to the optimal function of our bodies, providing required nutrients, excreting unwanted toxins and hormones, and ensuring a symbiotic relationship with the trillions of bacteria that we always live in conjunction with. Signaling to the gut via the VN is of highest importance to our well-being.

SUPPORTING LUNG FUNCTION

After the gut, the next most vulnerable area for toxins to enter the body is through our lungs. An average person takes between 20,000 to 25,000 breaths per day, but as Patrick McKeown shared in his book *The Oxygen Advantage*, there is a significant variation between the healthiest breathers and the unhealthiest. The key to making this work well for you is to become an efficient breather. The most efficient breathers take 10–12 breaths per minute, while the least efficient can take between 18–20 breaths per minute.

As we know, the less efficient your breathing ability (and the lower your CO_2 tolerance), the more you will be in a sympathetic state. This primes your macrophages and innate immune cells to remain in an inflammatory "fight" state. When it comes to the lungs, the issue that will occur here is that the lack of parasympathetic VN signals, coupled with airborne inflammatory triggers, drives us to have inefficient breathing due to poor lung function.

Optimal lung function allows for efficient exchange of carbon dioxide for oxygen, enabling our red blood cells to offload carbon and onboard oxygen and take it around the body for each of our cells to access. The blood is pumped by the heart through the blood vessels, and the effectiveness of the gas exchange depends on the state of the body.

In a sympathetic state, the amount of oxygen is increased in the lungs due to mouth breathing and shorter, shallower breaths. At the same time, the heart rate increases, and the blood vessels constrict, increasing blood pressure and allowing for faster blood flow to the muscles. This is a beneficial tool in the short term or in short bursts but is terrible for our health if this state remains in the long term. This is because our bodies will remain in a stressed state and allow for sympathetic inflammatory activation of macrophages, including the alveolar macrophages in the lungs.

In a parasympathetic state with effective VN signaling, we breathe through our nose, allowing air to be filtered and not have to contend with as many inhaled particulate matter or airborne microbes. We will take slower, deeper breaths that are prompted through diaphragmatic contraction (run through the phrenic nerve, not the vagus nerve).

Most importantly, studies conducted as far back as 1963 have shown that a cut vagus nerve results in decreased lung volume and made gas exchange more difficult, causing a change in breathing pattern. Stimulation of the VN has shown a near immediate improvement in lung function, a slowing of the breath rate, and improved lung volume, as well as a greater efficiency in gas exchange. There are numerous studies on electrical vagus nerve stimulation as a promising therapy in asthma, COPD, and the breathing challenges of anaphylaxis.

The VN sends signals directly to the alveolar macrophages, which when functioning properly, are able to limit the inflammatory effects of these cells and ensure that the lungs remain patent and functional. A dysfunctional VN will not be able to keep these macrophages and other immune cells in check, allowing them to increase inflammatory cytokine release and causing a severe, rapid, and potentially life-threatening effect on lung function.

Alveolar macrophages are the first line of defense against pollutants and microbes that are inspired into the lungs. The autonomic driven state of these macrophages is of very high importance as inflammatory activated, fight-ready (M1) macrophages will react more severely than homeostatic, housekeeping (M2) macrophages. The state of these cells is directly linked to the autonomic signaling provided by the sympathetic nerves and the VN for parasympathetic activity.

Electrical vagus nerve stimulation is an effective treatment in acute respiratory distress syndrome, asthma, and even COVID-19-related breathing issues. It works by signaling through the VN to the STAT3 pathway of the alveolar macrophages, pushing them into an M2, homeostatic state and limiting the amount of inflammatory signaling that these cells will produce.

Learning to breathe efficiently and effectively is the best way to send a positive parasympathetic signal through your body and to upgrade the function of your vagus nerve.

DETOXIFICATION/ BIOTRANSFORMATION SYSTEM

"Detox" is a phrase that I believe is thrown around too easily, especially on social media. Doing a seven-day detox is not the same as a constantly functioning detoxification system within the body, coordinated by the VN and involving multiple organs including the liver and kidneys. Here is a simplified way to think of detoxification, and how the vagus nerve works to manage the biotransformation system.

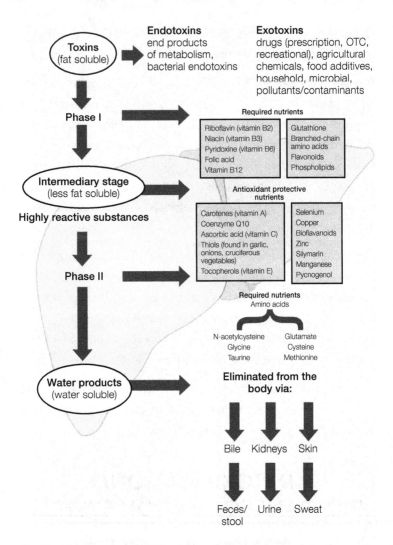

Toxins (fat soluble)

Endotoxins end products of metabolism, bacterial endotoxins

Exotoxins drugs (prescription, OTC, recreational), agricultural chemicals, food additives, household, microbial, pollutants/contaminants

Phase I

Required nutrients

Riboflavin (vitamin B2)
Niacin (vitamin B3)
Pyridoxine (vitamin B6)
Folic acid
Vitamin B12

Glutathione
Branched-chain amino acids
Flavonoids
Phospholipids

Intermediary stage (less fat soluble)

Antioxidant protective nutrients

Highly reactive substances

Carotenes (vitamin A)
Coenzyme Q10
Ascorbic acid (vitamin C)
Thiols (found in garlic, onions, cruciferous vegetables)
Tocopherols (vitamin E)

Selenium
Copper
Bioflavanoids
Zinc
Silymarin
Manganese
Pycnogenol

Phase II

Required nutrients
Amino acids

N-acetylcysteine
Glycine
Taurine

Glutamate
Cysteine
Methionine

Water products (water soluble)

Eliminated from the body via:

Bile   Kidneys   Skin

Feces/stool   Urine   Sweat

The liver has nearly 500 different functions and is the main biotransformation organ of the human body. The most important among these functions is the filtration of the portal veins and the biotransformation of toxic or inflammatory substances in the body. Once food has entered the digestive tract and has been digested and absorbed, it goes into the portal system, which are blood vessels that direct the digested products to the liver first. In the liver, the portal blood is filtered to ensure that unwanted toxins do not pass by and make their way to tissues that are incapable of handling them.

Within the liver, these toxins are then broken down in a two-phase process called "biotransformation," in which fat-soluble toxins are made more water soluble and released from the body in a third phase, via the stool, urine, and sweat. These pathways are outlined in the image on page 118.

BLOOD PRESSURE MANAGEMENT

Blood pressure (BP) is measured in two important areas by the VN. These are in the carotid artery and aorta by the use of carotid and aortic baroreceptors, which are neuronal receptors found in the lining of the blood vessels. They are constantly monitoring the flow of blood as well as the resilience of the vessel walls to maintain, constrict, or dilate their diameter to accommodate the blood flow through the vessel.

Afferent information on the flow state of blood through the vessels is relayed to the CNS via the VN, and determinations are made on a constant basis about whether to send a signal of constriction or dilation to the blood vessels. Other efferent signals are sent to the kidneys to manage the quantity of fluid and electrolytes in the body.

The role of the kidney is to filter blood to eliminate toxins while ensuring the optimal balance of fluid and electrolytes in the bloodstream. Within the kidney, there are systems of tubules and filters that send in and out water, sodium, potassium, calcium, chloride, and magnesium to form urine and manage our level of hydration.

Hydration level is highly involved in blood pressure maintenance. The VN carries efferent signals to the kidney to manage the blood flow and blood pressure through these organs.

AFFERENT FUNCTIONS IN THE CNS

Most of these functions are outlined in the anatomy section, in which we looked through the internal neuronal tracts of the CNS that move information from the NTS to the LC and all the adjacent nuclei to help with neuromodulation.

The optimization of neurotransmitter levels, signals of inflammatory control, and neuroplasticity through microglial management are relayed into the CNS via the VN, not exclusively, but it is a major component. When the VN is either not working or under significant distress, signaling in the CNS can become compromised and dysfunctional, resulting in low levels of inflammatory control and suboptimal neurotransmitter balance—a known cause of depression, anxiety, and PTSD.

INTEROCEPTION

As we previously have discussed, approximately 80 percent of all information carried on the VN is afferent, meaning it is going from the body to the brain. One of the most important reasons for the vast amount of status updates to the CNS is to create awareness and perception of the internal body functions and sensations—this is called "interoception." Interoception is like a sixth sense in that it allows us to sense and interpret signals from within our body and determine if things are functioning well or not.

We have all experienced sensations from within our bodies telling us that something just isn't correct. We may feel that our heart is pounding, our gut is feeling off for some reason, that we are breathing too heavily, or that our body temperature is changing.

When we turn our attention or awareness to what is happening inside our bodies, there are several specific components to interoception that we may notice changing, which are signaled through the VN.

◆ **Heartbeat and cardiac information:** We can sense changes to our heart rate and the quality of our heartbeat.

◆ **Gastrointestinal:** Our perception of hunger, fullness, digestive discomfort, and even motility challenges can be experienced by those with effective interoception.

◆ **Breathing and respiratory:** Bringing our awareness to the current state of our breath allows us to note breath rate, depth, and quality.

◆ **Emotional regulation:** The feeling of butterflies in your tummy before doing a presentation or the warmth that your body experiences when you lock eyes with an attractive person are all interoceptive feedback feelings of physiological changes linked to emotions. Emotions are experienced in physiological ways through interoceptive feedback. This is precisely how VN activity can influence our perception of stress, anxiety, and other emotions. Interoception makes up the practical component of mind-body connection.

◆ **Homeostasis and allostasis:** Allostasis is the measure of your body's ability to maintain stability (homeostasis) or optimal function in the face of stressors. Allostasis allows your body to cope with acute challenges and continue to function relatively well. In order to remain in a functional state, constant relays of status information must be presented to the CNS, so it may coordinate the response to the stressors.

◆ **Recent studies at various institutions have brought awareness to the importance of interoception and its link to mental health dysfunction.** Interoceptive capacity tends to be diminished in those suffering from the following conditions:

△ **Depressive disorders:** In depressive disorders, there tends to be a reduced awareness of bodily sensations, including hunger, fatigue, satiety, and pain, which can contribute to the neglecting of self-care and cause worsening symptoms.

△ **Anxiety disorders:** Hypersensitivity of interoceptive measures is often a characterization of anxiety disorders, leading to misinterpretation of these sensations as signs of threat of danger.

△ **Eating disorders:** Conditions such as anorexia nervosa and bulimia nervosa can involve atypical or distorted interoceptive processing related to hunger, fullness, and body image.

△ **Autism spectrum disorder (ASD):** Emotional dysregulation, lack of self-awareness, and difficulty with social interactions are keystone markers of ASD, linked to atypical interoceptive processing.

△ **Post-traumatic stress disorder (PTSD):** Hyperarousal and hypervigilance are major markers of PTSD, which is linked to internal sensations triggering potential traumatic memories and increased emotional distress.

△ **Somatization disorder:** Similar to PTSD, dysfunctional interoception may contribute to the perception of physical symptoms that are rooted in psychological distress.

△ **Body dysmorphic disorder:** An intense focus on perceived flaws in appearance may be related to atypical interoceptive processing and body image challenges.

△ **Panic disorder:** Interoceptive sensations of increased heart rate, shortness of breath, and sweating can be misinterpreted as signs of imminent danger, triggering a panic response.

Optimal interoception is an important piece to the health puzzle and is heavily associated with the perception of changes in bodily sensations being linked to emotional or psychological trauma. Interoception through the VN truly is the path of the mind-body connection.

CHAPTER 13

MEASURING VAGUS NERVE FUNCTION

When we want to drive to a new place, most of us will take out our phone, open a GPS-enabled app, and input the destination address or name of the business. The GPS application requires two pieces of information from you. First, it needs to know where you are currently located, and second, it needs to know where you want to go. The application will then provide detailed directions as to the current traffic conditions and the best routes to follow to reach the destination. The nuances of the route can be determined after, but the initial inputs required are the current and destination locations. Without these two pieces of information, the GPS app will not be of great value to you.

In the exact same manner, to take on the task of upgrading your vagus nerve, you must first become aware of its current functional status and second of your health goals with regard to vagus nerve function.

There are a few methods that enable us to assess the current function of our vagus nerve, as well as our progress. In this chapter we will go through the most important methods we have for assessing status as well as to track our progress as we move toward the goal of optimal health.

HEART RATE VARIABILITY

The single best metric when it comes to assessing VN and autonomic nervous system function is heart rate variability. Over the past decade, significant progress has been achieved by technology companies to make this metric much more accessible to us. HRV is the gold-standard metric, but we need to fully understand what it means and how to use this important data point to assess and track our progress.

What is heart rate variability (HRV) and what does it mean?

HRV is the ultimate measure of your body's adaptive capacity and resilience to challenge or stress, specifically regarding the function of the autonomic nervous system.

HRV provides insights into the dynamic interplay between the sympathetic and parasympathetic branches of the ANS and reflects the ability of the body to respond and adapt to internal and external stressors.

A healthy heart does not beat at a constant rhythm, but it rather exhibits slight variations in the time intervals between each heartbeat. These variations create a pattern known as HRV. The interval between successive heartbeats is influenced by various factors such as respiration, physical activity, emotions, and hormonal changes.

HRV analysis involves measuring the duration between successive R waves on an electrocardiogram (ECG) and extracting key parameters that describe the variability. These parameters include time-domain measures (e.g., standard deviation of normal-to-normal intervals) and frequency-domain measures (e.g., high-frequency power and low-frequency power).

Higher HRV is generally associated with better health and increased resilience. It signifies a well-functioning ANS with flexible and adaptive responses to different situations. Conversely, reduced HRV is often linked to various health conditions, including cardiovascular diseases, stress, anxiety, and autonomic dysfunctions.

Let's look at an example to ensure that we all understand how HRV is measured, going forward. To do this, we can compare two individuals with the same heart rate, measured in beats per minute.

When we measure the amount of time between R spikes (neural signals to the heart prompting a heartbeat), and we compare the average differences between these intervals over a period of time, we get a measure known as HRV.

Person A has a higher degree of variability in the number of milliseconds between successive beats. Person B has a lower degree of variability in the number of milliseconds between successive beats. Person B's heart beats more like a metronome, meaning that Person B doesn't have variation in the signals coming from sympathetic nerves sending norepinephrine and parasympathetic nerves sending acetylcholine. The lack of variability between these signals leads to less adaptive capacity and lower resilience. Person A has a higher HRV and is more adaptable. Person B has a lower HRV and is less adaptable to stressors.

Parasympathetic signals from the VN are meant to slow down the heartbeat by elongating the time between successive beats. Sympathetic signals are working to speed up the heart rate by decreasing the time between successive beats.

The optimal goal is a high degree of balance between parasympathetic and sympathetic. The analogy of the accelerator and brakes of a car are valuable here. A car is useless if only the brakes can be pushed and the accelerator doesn't work. The same car with ineffective brakes and a highly effective accelerator is a danger to others around it. The optimal function of a car is to have an effective accelerator and an effective functional brake pedal. A car needs to speed up to get moving and slow down to ensure the safety of those around. In the same way, the human body needs to be able to start up and get moving when there is a challenge to overcome or a threat to defend against, but it also requires the effective ability to slow, stop, and recover when there are no threats to act against.

In this exact way, a heart that beats more regularly, almost like a metronome, is mostly receiving information from sympathetic inputs, like a car whose driver is constantly pushing on the accelerator. As such, the variations in interbeat intervals will become less irregular and act as a sign that there are greater sympathetic signals coming to the heart than parasympathetic signals. This leads to low variability and is a sign of imbalance between sympathetic and parasympathetic inputs.

The alternate case is one in which the sympathetic and parasympathetic signals are relatively equal and strong. This scenario will lead to a greater amount of variability in the number of milliseconds between beats of the heart. The time between each beat will differ more substantially, as the signals from parasympathetic (brakes) and sympathetic (accelerator) are equal and able to get you moving when you need to, but allow you to slow down and recover when you need to. This is the definition of being adaptable and resilient.

Much new research is being completed, but current research has conclusively shown that higher HRV is associated with:

- **Lower risk of cardiovascular diseases:** Higher HRV indicates better heart health and a lower risk of heart-related issues, such as hypertension and heart attacks.
- **Improved emotional well-being:** Individuals with higher HRV tend to experience less anxiety and stress and have better emotional regulation.
- **Enhanced exercise performance:** Higher HRV is associated with better physical fitness and improved exercise capacity.
- **Better recovery from illness and injury:** A robust ANS response supports the body's ability to recover from illnesses and injuries more effectively.

One of my mentors, Ben Pakulski, a former elite-level body-builder and current host of the *Muscle Intelligence Podcast*, had a great, subjective way to measure your adaptability. He asked us to consider the following scenario: If you were sitting at a desk working, how quickly would your body be able to adapt to get up and sprint for 60 seconds (sympathetic drive)? And once you were able to complete the 60-second sprint, how easy would it be for your body to sit down and adjust back to a calm, relaxed recovery state (parasympathetic drive)?

There are three potential patterns that can give us an indication of your adaptability:

Pattern 1: If you are capable of getting up quickly and sprinting without much issue, then your sympathetic activation is effective, and you are relatively capable of sitting down and getting reset in front of the computer quickly following that sprint. This is an ideal pattern that indicates sympathetic and parasympathetic branches of the ANS are both functioning effectively. You will likely have a higher HRV, as you are highly adaptable and resilient to the challenge set out.

Pattern 2: Your body is slow and unable to get up and go for that sprint quickly. Essentially your body is not as adaptable to higher stress, but you are capable of sitting back down at your desk and getting back to work quite quickly. This is a sign of sympathetic deficiency and parasympathetic efficiency. This is the least common scenario and often will have a lower HRV finding.

Pattern 3: Your body is relatively quick to get up and go for the sprint, but significantly slower to adapt to a recovery state following the sprint, experienced by taking a long time to get your breath to slow down and your attention to focus back on the work. This is a sign of sympathetic efficiency and parasympathetic deficiency. This is the most common in my clients and patient population; this finding is directly linked to VN dysfunction. This person will often have a lower HRV.

The higher your HRV, the more adaptable you are to challenge and stress because you have greater ability to turn on sympathetic nerves when you need them and to turn on parasympathetic signaling via the VN when you need it.

NUANCE IN UNDERSTANDING AND USING HRV DATA

There is important nuance within the measurement and comparison of heart rate variability. First, no two people are the same, and HRV measurement compared between individuals should never be done. Please never make decisions about your health simply by comparing your HRV to another person's.

An individual's HRV can be highly variable from day to day or even minute to minute. Your HRV measurement will differ based on foods you have eaten, quality of sleep, current breathing patterns, blood sugar levels, exercise and movement, and any number of other variables. As such, the goal with HRV measurement should simply be to get the number higher than your personal baseline average on a daily basis.

Dr. Mike T. Nelson, a renowned exercise physiologist and guru in the HRV space, is a strong proponent of using a single HRV measure each morning within five to ten minutes of waking up daily. Depending on the wearable device you are using, this is a tool that can be measured in anywhere between one and five minutes each morning at approximately the same time. By assessing your HRV in this short measurement each morning, you will be given a number that accurately reflects your body's current state of recovery and ability to challenge yourself or take on new stressors effectively.

Many athletes use this exact method to assess their daily capacity to train and recover. As HRV is a measure of adaptability, the higher the HRV, the more adaptable they will be to take on greater training challenge as well as greater ability to recover from said challenge. A lower HRV is used as a sign not to push yourself quite so hard during that daily training session, as the body is not as adaptable on that particular day.

WHAT ARE THE BEST HRV MEASUREMENT DEVICES?

When it comes to using wearable devices to track HRV, there are two very important caveats to share. First, you should never directly compare the data from different devices to one another. They all use different sensors, different algorithms, and different forms of measurement. Once you choose a single device, keep consistent with the use of that device and do not compare it directly with another, as the numbers are likely to be different. Second, be aware that any wearable device should never be used for diagnostic purposes. These devices should only be used for tracking purposes, specifically for noting trends in a positive or negative direction compared with baseline or average values. This is an important disclaimer!

The gold standard for HRV measurement is without a doubt a medical-grade ECG device that is found primarily in medical clinics. These devices are wonderful for accurate measurements and great when used in a diagnostic setting. The difficulty is that these devices are not easy to wear, accessible, or readily available to the public. This is where wearable health-tracking devices can fill a need to understand our current and long-term health status.

The most accurate wearable devices for measuring HRV tend to be chest-strap devices that measure the electrical activity of the heart. As I am writing this, the Polar H10 or Biostrap Chest Strap are two amazing choices for this form of measurement. As accurate as they are, they can be a little difficult to put on and take off all the time and can be annoying to wear on your chest during a workout. They are also not intended to be worn for a longer time, such as through the night. If you are solely interested in accurate HRV measurements daily for a few minutes or to track heart rate through a workout, these are very good options.

Some of the more common devices on the market are wrist based and often are included as a measurement tool on a watch or other device. Fitbit and Garmin devices are quite good as health trackers and have relatively high accuracy when it comes to HRV-specific measurement.

Apple Watch and Samsung Smartwatch are very common devices that don't have the highest accuracy for HRV measurement but are pretty good when it comes to overall fitness tracking. The good news is that they can update their algorithms and have a massive amount of data coming into their systems due to the sheer quantity of users. This will allow for accuracy to increase in the coming months and years, which should be of great value to users of these devices.

Wrist-based health, fitness, and training devices are actually very accurate and have wonderful data inputs and outputs for their users. My favorite options in this category are Whoop and Biostrap wristbands. They use photoplethysmography (PPG) measurements to track the pumping of blood through blood vessels in the wrist. These tend to be the preferred choice of those seeking support with athletic endeavors and training.

One of my personal favorite devices is the Oura Ring. As of now I have had my Oura for nearly five years and love the data I get from it. It is a ring that fits on your finger and has a relatively high accuracy for HRV and exercise tracking, but its strength lies in accurate sleep measurements. The only issue with this type of device is that I do need to remove it while lifting weights or playing golf—any exercises that involves use of the hands for gripping— as the ring can become scratched or can be uncomfortable while gripping due to its thickness.

I am happy to share my top recommendations here, but remember that we are in the health-technology age, and this information is likely to become dated in the very near future with lots of new technology always becoming available.

HEART RATE RECOVERY

This is the measurement tool alluded to in the "Heart Rate Control" section on page 108. Heart rate recovery (HRR) is the measurement in the difference in beats per minute from the time that exercise ended and one minute following the end of the exercise. This measurement is dependent on a couple of factors: age and maximal heart rate during exercise. As we age, our HRR will naturally lower and tends to be minimal after the age of 60.

The only way to accurately measure this is to have a heart rate measurement wearable device (it doesn't need to be able to measure HRV for this test). To perform this test, measure your heart rate immediately at the end of your workout, and then again exactly one minute later. If your heart rate at the end of your workout is 150 bpm, and your heart rate one minute later is 130 bpm, then your HRR value is 20 bpm.

A study from the *New England Journal of Medicine* in 1999 found that a lower HRR value was linked to a higher rate of mortality and was attributed to lower vagal signaling. An average HRR was around 17 bpm (25th to 75th percentile values were 12–23 bpm) with elite male athletes having HRR scores of over 29 bpm. The concerning values were lower than 12 bpm, but the goal should be around 20 bpm lower at the one-minute mark than at the end of your workout.[12]

HRR values vary between individuals as well as from day to day. The goal for each person should simply be to get slightly better every day—to beat your average score each day and then to increase your average score over time.

If you are interested in improving this score, one of the best ways to do so is to learn to perform an active recovery at the end of your workouts. Most people will simply end a workout by immediately going back to the locker room or jumping in the shower without any time provided for active recovery. This is low-hanging fruit and a great time to practice improving vagal tone. Active recovery involves mindfulness practice immediately following the end of your workout for five to ten minutes in which you practice slow diaphragmatic breathing in a calm space. When done regularly, active recovery practice is one of the best ways to activate and improve vagus nerve function, as you will actively be learning to shift your state from sympathetic to parasympathetic. Active recovery practice will be discussed in Section 3 of this book.

PALATINE-ARCH RESPONSE— THE SAYING "AHH" TEST

As we have learned, contrary to the unique naming mechanism of calling it the vagus *nerve*, there are actually two vagus nerves, one protruding from each side of the brain stem at the medulla oblongata. These two nerves remain separate from one another until they enter the thorax and become intertwined, meshing together and coursing together along the esophagus and trachea and through the remainder of the thorax and abdomen. There is one area where we can perform a very simple test to see if one of the vagus nerves is more affected than the other—the soft palate.

When we swallow or speak, our soft palate (aka "velum"), the mucosal and muscular tissue located on the back end of the roof of our mouth, actually moves as well.

During swallowing, the soft palate elevates to seal off the nasopharynx from the oral cavity and prevent food or liquid from entering the nasal cavity. This movement is essential to ensure that the bolus (the chewed food mixed with saliva) travels down the esophagus and into the stomach without causing aspiration (inhalation of food or liquid into the respiratory tract). The elevation of the soft palate creates a physical barrier, directing the swallowed material downward and allowing it to pass safely through the upper respiratory and digestive tracts.

During speech production, the soft palate also elevates, but for a different reason. When we speak, air passes from the lungs through the trachea, and then through the vocal cords in the larynx, creating sound. The sound is then shaped into recognizable speech components by the movement of various articulators, including the tongue, lips, and soft palate.

Elevation of the soft palate during speech serves two purposes. First, it helps to create a pressure buildup in the oral cavity, necessary for producing certain speech sounds. When the soft palate is elevated, it blocks airflow through the nasal cavity, directing the air solely through the mouth for these specific speech sounds. Second, it prevents nasalization of non-nasal speech sounds. Nasalization occurs when the soft palate is not fully elevated, allowing some of the airflow to escape through the nasal cavity. Nasalization is appropriate for nasal speech sounds like /m/, /n/, and /ng/, but for other speech sounds, such as vowels and most consonants, it is undesirable.

An often-missed sign of VN dysfunction that is linked to this information is excessively nasal vocalization of sounds that should not have a nasal quality to them. When I work with clients, I not only listen to the words they are using but also the quality of their vocalization sounds, including nasal qualities and monotony, which are linked to the laryngeal branches of VN being negatively affected.

The palatine arches, which we can see when we look at the back of our oral cavity in the mirror (with the aid of effectively directed light), are innervated by two nerves—the pharyngeal branch of the vagus nerve supplying motor inputs to the muscles of the pharyngeal arches, and the lesser palatine nerves (monitoring sensory information), which are branches of the maxillary nerve, the fifth cranial nerve.

The ability to elevate the soft palate during swallowing and speech is directly linked to the effective function of the vagus nerve innervating the muscles of the palatine arches. The muscles of the left palatine arch are innervated by the pharyngeal branch of the left VN, and the muscles of the right palatine arch are innervated by the pharyngeal branch of the right VN.

The palatine-arch response test is a very simple test that anyone can perform on a daily basis. In order to perform this test, I recommend using a toothbrush (if you are performing the test at home) or tongue depressor (in a medical setting) to push down on your tongue, giving you a clear view of the palatine arches and uvula at the back of your throat.

While keeping your tongue depressed, look at the uvula protruding downward in the midline and the two arches directly adjacent to the uvula. Once you see these structures clearly, watch for the movement response they make when you say "Ahh."

An optimal response to this vocalization involves the following observations:

1. The left and right palatine arches elevate by approximately 1 cm (0.4 inches).
2. The arches elevate symmetrically when comparing them side by side.

3. The uvula elevates equally and remains in the midline of the body.

The movements to look out for as being less than optimal are as follows:

1. The palatine arches do not rise, or they elevate less than 1 cm.

2. The left and right palatine arches do not elevate symmetrically (one side elevates more than the other).

3. The uvula does not remain in the midline and begins to point to one side.

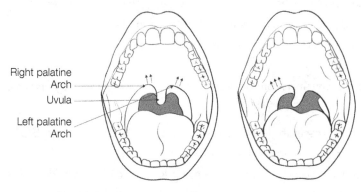

Asymmetric elevation of the arches will often result in combination with deviation of the uvula. If the left-side arch elevates more than the right side, then the uvula will deviate to point to the left side. The rule of thumb here is to note that the uvula will point to the side that is elevating more effectively. The uvula points to the side of VN that is working properly and away from the side that is not working as effectively.

We will often find major changes and deviations following physical traumas such as motor-vehicle accidents or slip-and-fall injuries due to the mechanism of injury affecting the brain stem negatively. Looking for minor variations and deviations on a regular basis can help to identify if there are suboptimal changes occurring between the two vagus nerves.

The palatine arch test will come in very handy when we look at vagus nerve stimulation and if there are any differences between stimulating on the left vs. right sides of the neck.

BOLT SCORE

The breath is the ultimate control mechanism by which we dictate to our body what state we want to be in. There is no better way to shift your autonomic state between sympathetic and parasympathetic than to control your breath.

Either your mind controls your breath, or your breath controls your mind.

In my research, I have yet to find a test better than the BOLT score to measure one's cardiovascular and biochemical capacity to remain resilient to the rising level of carbon dioxide. I was introduced to this test by Patrick McKeown in his book *The Oxygen Advantage*, and I have used this test with many of my clients with a high degree of success.

BOLT stands for "body oxygen level test." This simple test aims to measure the breath-holding time as an indicator of your tolerance to carbon dioxide (CO_2) and overall respiratory fitness.

Here's how the BOLT test is performed:

1. Preparation: Find a comfortable and quiet place to sit or lie down. Ensure that your posture is relaxed, with your spine straight and shoulders relaxed.

2. Take a normal breath: Breathe in and out through your nose a few times to settle into a calm and steady breathing pattern.

3. Empty your lungs: Take a normal breath in through your nose and then gently exhale all the air out through your nose. Completely empty your lungs and try to avoid any excessive breath-holding after the exhale.

4. Start the timer: After emptying your lungs, pinch your nose shut with your fingers (to avoid inhaling) and start the timer.

5. Hold your breath: Hold your breath for as long as you can, without straining or pushing yourself too hard. Focus on being relaxed during the breath hold.

6. End the test: When you feel the first involuntary need to breathe (i.e., when your body sends a signal that you need to take a breath), release your nose and breathe in gently through your nose. Note the time on the timer.

7. Calculate the BOLT score: The number of seconds you were able to hold your breath without the initial feeling of needing to inhale is your BOLT score.

Your BOLT score is a great way to assess your respiratory capacity on a weekly basis. Your BOLT score is something you can change for the better and is a test that points to overall respiratory efficiency as well as tolerance to rising CO_2 levels.

Here is what your BOLT score means:

A BOLT score of less than 10 seconds is a sign of poor cardiovascular capacity, chronic over-breathing, inefficient breathing mechanics, and potential respiratory issues.

A BOLT score between 10 and 19 seconds is a sign of inefficient breathing mechanics and lower cardiovascular capacity with low tolerance to CO_2 levels.

A BOLT score between 20 and 39 seconds is typical, representing average cardiovascular capacity, breathing mechanics, and moderate CO_2 tolerance.

A BOLT score of 40+ seconds is considered excellent, representing high CO_2 tolerance, optimal cardiovascular capacity, and optimal breathing mechanics.[13]

As we clearly know at this time, your BOLT score is not a direct marker of VN function; it is, however, a great surrogate marker to help determine respiratory efficiency and the biochemical capacity to handle higher levels of carbon dioxide. Within the 80 percent of afferent parasympathetic information carried along VN to the brain stem, there is status data from peripheral chemoreceptors found in the aortic body and carotid sinus that sense changes to blood CO_2 levels, oxygen levels, and acid-base balance (pH).

Contrary to popular belief, our respiratory efficiency is not linked to oxygen levels but rather carbon dioxide levels. The primary driver to take a breath is not to pull in more oxygen but to get rid of excess carbon dioxide.

As Patrick McKeown explains, carbon dioxide is the doorway through which we are able to get oxygen to reach our muscles. If the doorway is only slightly open, we will gasp for air more commonly (especially during exercise, but this can also happen at rest). If the doorway is wide open, we become more efficient at bringing oxygen into the cells. Chronic hyperventilation is the result of having a lower threshold to rising carbon dioxide levels. Efficient breathing patterns come from having a higher threshold to CO_2, or simply put, a higher CO_2 tolerance.

Chronic hyperventilation/over-breathing is linked to many health issues and activation of the sympathetic nervous system, including poor stress management, anxiety and mental health issues, poor sleep quality, lower exercise performance, poor cardiovascular health, and respiratory health conditions.

Effective control of breathing, particularly when we are not deliberately holding our breath, is by far the greatest lever by which we can affect autonomic state and function. If you truly want to work on upgrading your VN function, learning to breathe efficiently should be at the top of your daily practices.

BOWEL TRANSIT TIME TEST

This is a test that I shared in my previous book; however, it is very helpful to understanding the gastrointestinal component of VN health.

As we know, the GI tract is inextricably linked to the vagus nerve, which physically makes up the microbiome-gut-brain axis. The signals of current GI status and microbial balance are sent through the VN to the brain for processing. We also have many signals being sent through the VN to the intestinal macrophages, dictating their capacity to deal with inflammatory signals and limiting the chronicity of the inflammatory triggers. Signals to the gut are also necessary to promote intestinal peristalsis and the migrating motor complex, the effective movement of food through the digestive tract.

The bowel transit time test is a simple way to assess the current function of your digestive tract, specifically the efficiency of the gut to extract nutrients from food and eliminate waste in a timely manner. Here are simple instructions for performing this test.

1. Purchase a small amount of white sesame seeds from a local bulk or grocery store. One tablespoon is usually sufficient. Ensure that you do not purchase black sesame seeds as they can be more difficult to visualize when completing this test.

2. Measure one tablespoon of white sesame seeds and pour the seeds into a glass of water.

3. Drink the glass of water, being sure not to chew the seeds.

4. Mark down the time of ingestion on a journal or piece of paper.

5. Remember that you are doing this test when you go to the bathroom for a bowel movement over the next few days.

6. Take a look in the bowl following your bowel movement to assess if you see any white sesame seeds in your stools.

7. Mark down the date and time when you begin to see the seeds in your stools. Continue to do this at each bowel movement until you no longer see the seeds in your stools.

Refer to the chart below to check which category your bowel transit time is currently in.

Time from Ingestion to Visualization	Category	Explanation
Less than 12 hours	Too Fast	Very fast and inefficient bowel transit time
12–18 hours	Fast-Normal	Fast BTT but within allowable range
18–24 hours	Optimal	Optimal bowel transit time
24–36 hours	Slow-Normal	Slow BTT but within allowable range
Greater than 36 hours	Too Slow	Very slow and inefficient bowel transit time

An optimal bowel transit time is a great and simple assessment tool for gut function and is associated with good signaling along the VN to and from the gut. Any deviation from the optimal category can be a sign of inefficient gut function and potential triggers for, or signs of, VN dysfunction. They can be associated with diagnoses of irritable bowel syndrome (IBS), small intestinal bacterial overgrowth (SIBO), small intestinal fungal overgrowth (SIFO), or inflammatory bowel disease.

Use the bowel transit time test as a preliminary measurement tool to determine if more testing may be necessary to further understand microbiome balance and intestinal function.

PERCEIVED STRESS INVENTORY—SOCIAL READJUSTMENT RATING SCALE (SRRS)

As a gentle reminder, not all stress is bad. Stress is more distressing to us based on our perception of the challenge. If we feel that we are able to cope or handle a stressor, it will actually help us to have a more positive outlook and perceive it as a positive challenge rather than a negative stressor. With this said, there is a cumulative effect of stress, both positive and negative, on our ability to withstand. Assessing the amount of emotional or psychological stress we have recently been under can help us understand how much positive challenge we should take on.

The Holmes-Rahe Stress Inventory (aka Social Readjustment Rating Scale or SRRS) is a well-known and well-studied tool in psychology and a great component in understanding the amount of stress we feel that we are under. This one-page subjective assessment of recent challenges in our life can be useful in providing an understanding of the cumulative stress we feel we are subject to.

We must note that this assessment completed on its own has some limitations that must be addressed. The data points assessed are highly subjective, and there is limited scope of what is being evaluated. There is a recency bias that is inherent in the test itself, as we are reviewing only events that have taken place in the year prior to performing the test. As such, we are unable to truly account for major life events or chronic stressors on this test. To lower the burden of these limitations, it can be very beneficial to have a life event timeline assessment done with a practitioner that can help to parse out the effects that various challenges have had on one's physiological capacity to cope.

This said, the Holmes-Rahe Stress Inventory is a great tool that can help us understand the likelihood of a potential physiological or health event in the near future based on the amount of stress one has accumulated in the year prior.

This assessment is performed by taking inventory of the stressors noted on the form, each of which has been assigned a numerical value based on how stressful it tends to be perceived to be. For example, the death of a spouse has a numerical value of 100 points, while a change in residence is valued at 20 points and a vacation is valued at 13 points.

As we add up all the stressors that one has experienced in the past year, we find a total score of perceived stress, which is linked to the risk of stress-induced health breakdown taking place in the next two years.

Score*	Meaning
Less than 150 points	A relatively low amount of life stress and minimal risk of stress-associated health breakdown.
150–300 points	Moderate amount of stress and a 50 percent chance of a stress-associated health breakdown over the next two years.
Greater than 300 points	A high amount of stress and an 80 percent risk of a stress-associated health breakdown over the next two years according to the Holmes-Rahe statistical prediction model.

* Source: https://pubmed.ncbi.nlm.nih.gov/6059863.

At my online clinic, Health Upgraded, we believe in completing a thorough assessment of each client to fully understand the time-line of events in their life, their mindset around how stressors are or have affected them in their life, as well as looking at all areas in which stressors can be triggering physiological effects within their body. Regular assessment of HRV, BOLT scores, palatine-arch testing, bowel transit time, as well as personal stress inventory, allows us to provide the best recommendations to help our clients understand their root causes and quantify their progress.

We believe that it is of utmost importance to have as full a picture and as broad an understanding as possible of the potential root causes of stress, so that we can help our clients to take positive strides in addressing these stressors, while working to upgrade the function of their vagus nerve, so they build resilience and adaptive capacity to challenges that will inevitably arise in the future.

STRATEGIES FOR UPGRADING THE VAGUS NERVE

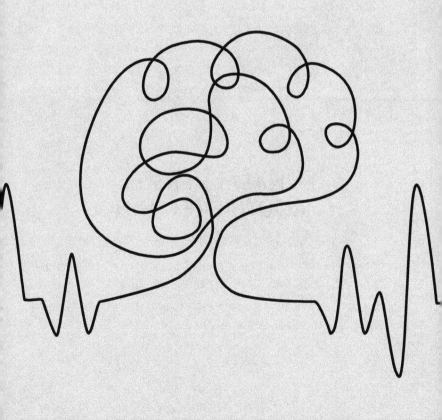

CHAPTER 14

BREATHING STRATEGIES

The importance and relevance of breath cannot be overstated when it comes to its effects on autonomic function and the VN specifically. Improper breathing patterns are the most pertinent piece of the therapeutic puzzle. Effective breathing can even be considered the linchpin for shifting one's state between sympathetic and parasympathetic, and this is why the following strategies are placed first in this section for upgrading the function of the vagus nerve.

NASAL VERSUS MOUTH BREATHING

Your nose is for breathing and your mouth is for eating. It truly is that simple, but fortunately we were designed with a backup plan in case the nose became blocked or dysfunctional. When we are at rest, we need to train ourselves to passively breathe through our nasal cavity by keeping our mouths closed.

As discussed in Chapter 4, addressing a deviated septum or the direct causes of nasal blockage is imperative to allowing you to use the nasal cavity as your primary breathing channel. Once the barrier to nasal breathing is addressed, it will become significantly easier to implement exercises to correct suboptimal patterns and habits.

If this is a challenge for you, a simple strategy to help is to close your mouth and place the tip of your tongue on the roof of your mouth just behind your two front incisors. You can use this strategy while initially making this change to your habits, and with regular work and reminders, this will become a positive passive habit.

INHALATION AND EXHALATION

An underutilized strategy in breathing exercises is to look at the ratio of time spent inhaling vs. exhaling. When we inhale, we send a signal to the body that we are under a bit of stress, and our body responds with a nominal but measurable elevation of our heart rate. This is countered during exhalation, as while we breathe out, the heart rate undergoes a nominal yet measurable decrease. Inhalation activates the sympathetic nerves, while exhalation activates the vagus nerve, having a parasympathetic effect on the heart. This is an impressive finding that we can strategize around to help rebuild our breathing patterns.

If the time spent inhaling is greater than the time spent exhaling, then we will tend to promote a sympathetic state more than a parasympathetic state.

This ratio is also highly relevant when it comes to our CO_2 tolerance and BOLT scores, as the primary driver and prompt for breathing is to release carbon dioxide from the body. If we have a lower tolerance to carbon dioxide levels, we will be prompted to exhale more quickly and more often. However, if we work to improve our tolerance to CO_2, then we can address and optimize this ratio.

To make the following practices a little easier, consider downloading a breath timer app that you can use to customize your own breath exercises.

A great beginner strategy for addressing the ratio is to practice the 4-4-4-4 box breathing method consisting of four-second inhalation, four-second hold, four-second exhalation, and again a four-second hold. This does not bring attention to a longer exhale time but does train the inhale-to-exhale ratio to become a 1-to-1 ratio, as many beginners often spend more time inhaling than exhaling.

The next level is to extend the exhale time and work toward doubling exhale time over inhale time. A simple tool for this is to practice the 4-4-6-2 breathing method of four-second inhale, four-second hold, six-second exhale, and two-second hold.

Once you feel confident with this practice, I like the 4-7-8 breathing method as a great top-end training tool. This strategy involves a four-second inhale, seven-second hold, and eight-second exhale.

A daily ten-minute breath-training practice session will eventually improve your passive inhale-exhale ratio and allow your body to have greater signaling capacity through the VN.

PHYSIOLOGICAL SIGHING

One unique strategy for acute elevations in parasympathetic activity is called the "physiological sigh." This involves the following pattern of inhalation and exhalation: Initially, take a relatively deep inhale, followed by a short but noticeable deeper inhale, then followed by a longer, fuller exhale. Simply put, you first breathe in, then quickly breathe in again, then slowly exhale and empty your lungs. The longer, slower exhale is particularly helpful in recruiting the parasympathetic response.

This seems to work by including the second inhale, which does two things. A second inhale is not normal in the breathing pattern, so it forces our attention to our breath. This in itself is great to help lower anxiety in the moment; however, on the physiological side, the second inhale seems to recruit less-utilized alveoli in the lungs, reengaging them and increasing the gas-exchange function by increasing lung surface area following the second inhale.

The physiological sigh is a tool that we can use in an acute situation of higher stress, such as feeling overwhelmed due to work or family commitments. Its practice does require you to become mindful of how you are feeling and when you are in need of a relaxation response. Sighing can be considered a respiratory reset for the body and is a great simple tool to help shift your state when you are feeling overwhelmed or stressed.

BREATH-HOLD TRAINING

Breath holding can have complex effects on the autonomic nervous system. The responses to breath holding vary based on the duration of breath holding, individual factors, and the specific context. Generally, the initial response to brief breath holding is sympathetic activation, followed by parasympathetic activation.

Initially, when you hold your breath, there is a buildup of carbon dioxide (CO_2) in the blood (called hypercapnia). This triggers a sympathetic response, leading to increased heart rate, increased blood pressure, and a sense of urgency. As breath holding continues, the CO_2 buildup becomes more pronounced, leading to a stronger stimulation of the parasympathetic nervous system. This parasympathetic response aims to restore balance and counteract the initial sympathetic activation. It slows down the heart rate, reduces blood pressure, and promotes relaxation.

The transition from sympathetic to parasympathetic dominance during breath holding reflects the body's attempt to maintain homeostasis. The parasympathetic response helps normalize the CO_2 levels in the blood and prevent an overly intense sympathetic response.

It's important to note that the balance between sympathetic and parasympathetic activation during breath holding can vary based on factors such as individual physiological differences, emotional state, and the duration of the breath holding.

Breath-hold training is an advanced-level tool to help upgrade the parasympathetic system and should only be used while being monitored by professionals. It is, however, one of the greatest tools for those looking to significantly improve their CO_2 tolerance and to train their ability to improve VN function and elevate HRV.

ACTIVE RECOVERY TRAINING

I was first introduced to this concept by a fitness coach working with Ben Pakulski and have been utilizing it with high efficacy and noticeable improvement in my recovery following my workouts.

Active recovery involves taking between five and ten minutes at the end of a workout to focus on actively breathing more slowly and shifting your state from sympathetic, at workout's end, to parasympathetic soon after the workout ends. As we know, the key to upgraded health is resilience to stress, so we need to make the recovery process as efficient as possible, increasing our resilience.

Hormesis is a biological phenomenon by which low to moderate exposure to a stressor results in a greater capacity to adapt and become resilient to the stressor. Exercise is a hormetic stressor, known to have significant positive health-adaptive responses. The active recovery process is key to improving resilience and helping to build efficiency in this adaptive capacity.

Following a workout, active recovery involves sitting or lying down for a short period of time, pulling your attention back to your breath, and actively slowing the breath rate while focusing on longer exhalations and diaphragmatic breathing. Completing between five and ten minutes of active recovery following your workouts is a very effective way to stimulate the vagus nerve and help your body build the necessary resilience to bounce back when encountering future stressors.

CHAPTER 15

NONINVASIVE ELECTRICAL VAGUS NERVE STIMULATION

If I had to choose a single therapy that I am most excited about and which has shown the greatest benefit to my clients over the last couple of years, the answer is, without a doubt, noninvasive electrical VNS.

I first introduced this technology into my practice when I was having some difficulty supporting my patients with the exercises and nutritional supplementation on their own. The issue was that these patients were hitting a plateau with their inability to shift state from sympathetic to parasympathetic. The technology was intriguing to me initially, but upon my trying the gammaCore cervical VNS device developed by Electrocore Inc., I became very excited to begin supporting my patients with this therapy... and it has not disappointed at all!

Electrical VN stimulation (VNS) was first attempted in the 1960s to treat epileptic seizures, and despite initially having inconsistent results, a study at the University of Alabama in 1988 success-fully found a method to perform VNS to reduce the frequency of seizures in epileptic patients. The FDA first approved implantable devices for epileptic patients in 1997. Over the subsequent decades, research has been done to find ways to bring this therapy to more people dealing with chronic health conditions by making the therapy noninvasive and highly effective.

The range of conditions that VNS has been tested for and has had very positive results in is quite dramatic—treatment-resistant depression, generalized anxiety, migraine headache, cluster headache, trigeminal neuralgia, gastroparesis, inflammatory bowel disease, irritable bowel disease, stroke, traumatic brain injury, post-traumatic stress disorder, Parkinson's disease, and Alzheimer's disease all being among the conditions cited thus far. There is a reason for this broad spectrum of conditions that have benefited from the use of this technology—the technology is not a cure for any particular condition at all, it is a device meant to help create a state shift.

Conventional medicine is focused on the pathway of symptoms and signs, testing to verify, and the declaration of a diagnosis, followed by using a single therapy to treat or manage the specific diagnosis. This methodology absolutely is effective and the best way to support patients dealing with an acute condition. In a chronic setting, however, this methodology is flawed.

Nearly all chronic lifestyle-based health conditions have a common pathway of uncontrolled inflammation. The cumulative effect of stressors, compounding over time paired with the reduced capacity to control the inflammatory reaction, will eventually lead to systemic breakdown and the diagnosis of a chronic disease. The underlying stressors push on the accelerator, while the brakes wear down over time, resulting in the inability to slow down the proverbial car.

VNS is a special therapy, as it is meant to drive the ability to control inflammation via the vagus nerve. It affects the parasympathetic nervous system and the cholinergic anti-inflammatory pathway directly, with the outcome being improved control of inflammation and immune cell activation. The use of electricity to achieve this reaction is highly effective. The use of VN exercises is necessary and foundational—breathing, gargling, gag reflex, cold exposure, social connectedness, and many other exercises are all important; however, they are often not strong enough on their own to create the required state shift and allow the body to recover effectively.

When a car has broken down, a mechanic needs to take a look under the hood and figure out the cause of the problem. This cannot be done if the car is in motion. If the accelerator is constantly being pushed, the mechanic can listen to the sounds and watch the motion of the car to assess what may be dysfunctional in the first place, but he/she will likely be incapable of fixing the problem while the car continues to move. We need to slow down and eventually stop the car so the problem can be fixed. The brakes need to work well enough for the mechanic to put it on the hoist or open the hood.

For many people suffering from chronic diseases, it is as though their brakes just aren't working, and they are truly unable to slow down to the point where repair and healing can occur.

Healing cannot take place in a sympathetic state.

The parasympathetic state is required for rest, digest, and RECOVERY.

VNS is a game-changing therapy that helps to push on the brakes and put the body into a parasympathetic state for some time, allowing the body to begin the healing process. Once my qualifying patients use this therapy, they will often notice that the nutritional, supplemental, and lifestyle strategies that we have implemented become much more effective, and the healing process can actually take place.

I will always choose a noninvasive therapy when given the opportunity. Devices that do not require surgical intervention are ideal when they have similar effectiveness, and that is why I am a fan of the use of electrical stimulation of the cervical trunk of VN within the neck. The therapies I choose for my clients are those that are easy to implement within their lives and have the minimum dose with the highest effectiveness.

The cervical trunk is the most easily accessed part of the VN— simply use your index and middle fingers to find your pulse in your neck, and you will be within a few millimeters of your vagus nerve. The VN is well protected within the carotid sheath but is accessible using electricity. There are a few muscles in the area that you should be aware of—platysma, which is very thin and overlies the entire front of the neck; sternocleidomastoid (SCM), which is the thick band lateral to the carotid sheath on both sides of the neck; and the anterior and middle scalenes are also located just deep to the SCM and carotid sheath. If you have difficulty finding your pulse, work with a healthcare practitioner to help you locate the area that you are looking for.

This therapy has been proven through fMRI studies to stimulate the nucleus of the solitary tract and create a biphasic response in the central nervous system that stimulates the parasympathetic nervous system while downregulating the sympathetic nervous system within 15 minutes of a two-minute stimulation.

One of the most exciting pieces of information regarding VNS that I have come across is its ability to upgrade cognition and learning speeds. A double-blind sham-controlled study done at the Defense Language Institute in Monterey, California—the US Department of Defense's premier language school—showed that VNS with the gammaCore device accelerated the learning of Arabic vocabulary by 25 percent. Participants in this study showed significant increases in energy and focus of the course of their training sessions compared to sham participants.[14]

In another study, the US Air Force found that after 34 hours of wakefulness (sleep deprivation in drone pilots), VNS with the gammaCore device allowed participants to perform significantly better on arousal and multitasking and reported significantly lower fatigue ratings when compared with sham. VNS has been found to be a powerful countermeasure to fatigue and supports the brain's ability to function at a higher level.[15]

CROSS-SECTION FRONT OF NECK C6
(Level of the 6th cervical vertebra)

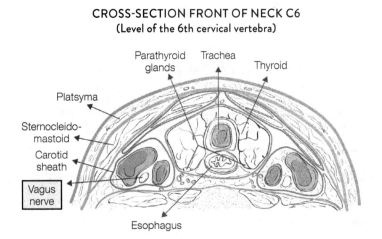

There are other therapies and devices on the market, but I have found VNS to be most easy to implement in short time spurts in the morning and evening with a small device that conveniently can fit in a pocket. People can easily travel with it and use it a couple times per day, as the effects last for anywhere between 12 to 48 hours. As a practitioner, my favorite device recommendation is the one that the client will be able to use as per my recommendations with the greatest regularity and consistency.

The most exciting part for me is that this therapy has minimal unintended side effects. Often I will hear that my patient is less stressed, more energetic, sleeping better, and able to take on a positive outlook, allowing them to handle stressors in a more positive and head-on manner. I will then pair this therapy with the nutritional, lifestyle, and stress management strategies in this book to create the best possible outcome and improve resilience to future challenges when working with my clients.

CHAPTER 16

NUTRITIONAL STRATEGIES

A significant and overlooked component of upgrading vagus nerve function is through optimizing nutrition. There are foods that we need to incorporate into our diets to supply raw materials for ACh production, as well as foods to exclude from our diets as they are common triggers to inflammation, acting as biochemical stressors that will alter the microbiome population and trigger hormonal and biochemical stress internally.

There is a significant amount of debate in the public sphere regarding specific diets—carnivore vs. animal-based vs. plant-based vs. vegan vs. vegetarian vs. paleo vs. keto vs. Mediterranean vs. pescatarian. I am not going to place myself into this debate as I do not feel that there is a single diet that has a positive effect on every single person. That said, there are some common threads among most of these diets that are observed and almost everyone can agree on due to the conclusive nature of research findings over the past few decades. I personally have tried versions of most of these diets, and I believe that each individual must determine what works for them personally. Be mindful, be aware, and learn to hear the whispers from your body if something is not working well or if you feel better with certain foods.

Signs that you are reacting poorly to a specific food can include any of the following: bloating or digestive distress, constipation, diarrhea, nasal stuffiness, low energy and sluggishness, sneezing, coughing, redness, hives or histamine reactions, skin itchiness or irritability, and elevated heart rate. These signs can occur immediately or slowly over a couple days after eating a particular food. Most people are unaware that a specific food is a trigger for these reactions, so using a food-and-symptom diary is a great idea for 3 to 14 days to help you determine if there is a potential dietary trigger.

COMMON TRIGGERING FOODS TO AVOID

First, we should discuss the foods that we need to avoid or eliminate, as they are common triggers to inflammation and biochemical stress. The common thread through this section will be foods that are highly processed. In general, the more a food is processed, the higher the calories and the lower the nutrient status of that food. Not to mention that many of these processed foods contain highly processed and inflammatory seed oils.

I highly recommend becoming an ingredient list reader when you are choosing what to bring home from the grocery story. Packaged foods with greater than five ingredients listed should be used minimally, as these are the main culprits of high-calorie, low-nutrient-density foods. Ingredients that everyone should look out for and avoid due to their inflammatory nature include: vegetable oil, canola oil, soybean oil, safflower oil, palm oil, palm kernel oil, margarine, high-fructose corn syrup, added sugars, artificial chemicals or additives, and MSG.

Some people have health challenges that can be triggered by specific foods as well, including gluten-containing grains, specifically wheat, barley, rye, and spelt. Others don't do well with dairy due to lactose sugar or casein protein. These people would do best to eliminate triggering foods and even the highly processed substitutes that tend to include excessive ingredients to mask their poor taste.

Processed meats are another area that we need to be careful of due to the use of nitrates, nitrites, or the curing process. These have been shown to cause some forms of cancer and need to be minimized or eliminated entirely from our diets. Conventionally raised meats tend to have a diet high in grains, which increases the amount of omega-6 fatty acids in their bodies, which are inflammatory for humans.

Frequently overlooked challenges for some (but not all) people are plant-defense chemicals, specifically tannins, saponins, isothiocyanates, lectins, and oxalates found in many plants, particularly leafy vegetables. These are found in the part that the plant doesn't want us to eat. We should be focused primarily on fruits, which are the part that the plant truly wants us to eat. Contrary to popular belief, kale, spinach, and tomatoes may cause harm to some people and should be assessed to determine if they may actually be doing more damage than good—this is, however, a very individual issue that needs to be scrutinized by you and a professional to determine the potential risk.

FOODS TO INCLUDE

The simple answer to the question "What should I eat" is WHOLE foods. This may be too simple an answer for some, but it is the absolute truth of the matter with resounding evidence. The general consensus is that the Mediterranean diet is the healthiest form of diet, which is a great starting point for most of us who are looking to improve our health in some way. From here we should refine and personalize the diet to exactly what works best for us individually.

The highest quality protein options include grass-fed, grass-finished beef; organic chicken or turkey; organic pork; wild-caught low-mercury fish; and hunted game meat—essentially animals raised without the use of hormones, additives, or chemicals, and fed an evolutionarily consistent diet are the best options to support protein intake.

When it comes to choline, organic eggs, particularly runny egg yolks, and organ meats are by far the highest sources of choline. For those who choose not to eat animal products, soybeans, potatoes, and quinoa are substitutes that do have some choline present, but it is significantly less absorbable and bioavailable (bioavailable refers to the effective absorption rate of a nutrient).

From the plant food side of the equation, focusing on organic fruits and vegetables is of highest importance while personalizing the choices to what your body can handle effectively. Although some vegetables are better when eaten raw, others ideally should be cooked. The benefit of vegetables is their fiber content. I personally prefer cooked vegetables, but this is something you need to test to determine the best options for you.

Fruits have been unfairly demonized and should be present in most diets. Fructose has been given a bit of a bad rap lately, but the reality is that the benefits of the lower carbohydrate content in fruit, as well as the antioxidants and bioflavonoids, far outweigh any negatives that can come from the low level of naturally occurring sugars in fruits. Personalize your choices here but know that fruit is actually very healthy and good for you. Try to choose locally grown and seasonal options to ensure that nutrient content is aligned with your geography.

SUPPLEMENTS TO CONSIDER

I am a proponent of getting your nutrients from your food first. If your diet is complete and full of whole foods, there will be minimal gaps in your nutrient intake. That said, the current reality is that most people don't have the best nutrition, and supplements can help to fill some of the gaps that seem to be missing. Nutritional supplements are (as their name indicates) supplemental and should not be thought of as the primary source of a nutrient unless there is a medical reason for doing so.

Here are my top five supplements for vagus nerve health:

1. A source of B vitamins: B vitamins are an absolute necessity for mitochondrial function and must be considered if your diet is less than ideal. B vitamins can be sourced from organ meat as well as plants, but they truly are one of the most overlooked and necessary options when it comes to optimizing mitochondrial health and energy levels in the body. B vitamins are included in many steps to create acetyl-CoA, which we know is necessary in the production of acetylcholine.

NMN (nicotinamide mononucleotide) and NR (nicotinamide riboside) are also great mitochondrial-supporting supplements that have shown improved energy and longevity biomarkers due to their ability to increase NAD+ levels.

2. A source of choline: As discussed in the biochemical stress section of the book, choline is deficient in 90 percent of diets. Most of us do not get enough at all, and the VN requires choline to be able to signal using ACh.

Choline supplementation can be confusing, as there are four main forms that it can be taken in—choline bitartrate and choline chloride, the salt forms, are not my favorites but are much more common. Alpha-GPC and phosphatidylcholine are my preferred sources of choline via supplementation due to their higher bioavail-ability and decreased elevation of TMAO (which we discussed in the nutrition/biochemical stress section). Sunflower lecithin is a great lower-cost plant-based source of phosphatidylcholine as well.

3. Anti-inflammatory supplements: Omega-3 fatty acids and turmeric are my top supplements to help lower inflammation within the body. Omega-3 sources such as fish oils are great to help bring the omega-3 to omega-6 ratio into a favorable balance. Turmeric is a well-known plant containing curcumin that has been used for many generations to lower inflammation through Ayurve-dic and traditional Chinese medicine practices.

4. Amino acids: As protein is often the macronutrient missing from our diet, we are not receiving an adequate quantity of amino acids. It may be because food choices are lacking in protein options, or that our digestive system is not functioning optimally to absorb the amino acids from the gut, but one of the most common findings in functional lab tests is a lack of these important building blocks.

If you test urinary organic acid levels using functional laboratory testing as many functional medicine practitioners do, then it may be easier to supplement specific amino acids such as glycine, gluta-mine, or n-acetyl cysteine; however, a full-spectrum amino acid powder can be beneficial for those who don't complete the testing. This is different from protein powder, as amino-acid supplements have been broken down into component "Lego blocks" and can be taken individually or in combination with one another, but they are far easier to absorb in this scenario.

5. Electrolytes: Supplementation with electrolytes has more to do with poor hydration practices than anything else. We have been told to drink eight glasses of water per day, but this doesn't restore everything we lose daily through water loss. Water is lost through the breath, urine, sweat, and stool, and it's often pulled out of the body with the flow of mineral salts or electrolytes.

Restoration of electrolyte levels in the body is imperative for optimal cellular function. This means we should be resupplying the necessary minerals back into our body with fluid intake. Sodium, potassium, magnesium, chloride, and calcium are the main elec-trolytes to add in, especially for those who sweat a lot or during/after any workout.

In my practice, I have found that supplements can be very benefi-cial to fill gaps in nutritional status, and that herbal therapeutics can be as effective as some medications. I am, however, very particular when it comes to making recommendations, as objective testing is often the best way to determine the specific gaps for each individ-ual. There is no single supplement that will fix all issues across the board. Allowing our bodies to get into a parasympathetic state will finally allow for nutrients to be absorbed, and ideally we can get the majority of our nutritional needs from dietary sources and simply fill the individual gaps with supplements.

CASE STUDY: SANDRA

Sandra was in the ICU with severe COVID in December 2021. It wasn't looking great for her. She had severe breathing issues, severe fatigue, and brain fog. Thankfully, the acute treatments provided by her healthcare team were powerful enough to bring her back from the brink, and she got out of the hospital with a renewed sense of direction and desire to get back to optimal health. She began trying different diets and interventions with quite terrible results.

Her story was marred with emotional and psychological stressors—a difficult childhood due to a poor relationship with her mother was at the root of her trauma; however, the significant challenge occurred when she lost her teenage son eight years prior in a tragic car accident for which she blamed herself, even though she was not involved at all.

Her downward spiral affected her health so badly that she gained a significant amount of weight over the years, feeling so ashamed that she wasn't comfortable even turning on the camera to join me on a Zoom call.

She had been diagnosed with type 2 diabetes as her hemoglobin A1C marker had gone up to 8.1 mmol/L while she was in the hospital for COVID and increased to 9.3 mmol/L following trying a vegan diet to help with her weight challenges. Her fasting glucose was consistently at 154 mg/dL when she first began working with us (ideal is between 80 to 100). Depression following her emotional stress was also quite evident. She was adamant about not wanting to use medication to address her HbA1C, until she had exhausted all natural remedies and options by working with us at Health Upgraded.

Sandra began her program with us using some functional lab testing, allowing us to identify nutritional deficiencies and microbiome imbalances. We helped her refine her diet to focus on high-quality protein intake, a couple of vegetables, and some mild fruit intake. We found a significantly low level of *Akkermansia muciniphila* bacteria in her microbiome testing, which was directly correlated, and we addressed it directly with targeted probiotic therapy. Lastly, Sandra also added vagus nerve stimulation with the gammaCore VNS device daily.

After a few months, we were excited about her progress—her mood had improved, her energy was better, her HbA1C was tested and had come down to 7.1 mmol/L (from 9.3), and her fasting glucose hovered between 95 to 116 mg/dL. She notes that feeling stressed absolutely drives her glucose levels up, and she was very happy with the VNS therapy.

This past year, on the anniversary of her son's passing, Sandra noticed something different. The emotional pain was still there, and still quite raw, but she noticed that she didn't have any heart palpitations, an issue that had come up for a few weeks around this date for the past eight years. This year, no palpitations were noted. She sent me a note saying: "The emotions and feelings are still there, my body just handled it differently. I feel like I'm finally healing. I just had to share that with you. Thank you so much!!!"

CHAPTER 17

AUDITORY/LISTENING THERAPY

In this chapter, we will review two major sources of therapy for the vagus nerve using sound. The first is vocalization featuring the use of our own vocal cords, and the second is auditory or listening therapies that involve the use of our sense of hearing.

VOCALIZATION—HUMMING, CHANTING, SINGING, GARGLING

As we know, the laryngeal muscles are innervated directly by the superior and inferior laryngeal branches of VN. Along with the pharyngeal branch of VN, these are the only efferent motor neuronal branches on this nerve. As such, the activation of the muscles around the vocal cords can be used very effectively to stimulate electrical activity along the VN. As we can only vocalize while we are exhaling, they do double duty in activating parasympathetic activity due to the necessity of the exhale being added to the activation of vocal cord laryngeal musculature.

In my previous book, I included many vocalization tools that I recommend to my clients due to their ability to support and improve VN function. Here I will review a few of the more effective and easier to implement vocalization exercises.

Humming is a relatively straightforward practice to include in your daily life and one that works well with children. I have two young daughters who are quite active, especially between the end of their school day and dinnertime in our home. Once it is time for us to sit at the table, we enter "digest" mode. Sometimes this will include some slow belly-breathing practices, and other times it involves humming for as long as we can. We pretend that we are buzzing like bees, getting ready to have our meal.

Chanting is a practice that has been around for thousands of years—from the "om" recitation during meditation practice in the Hindu tradition to Gregorian chanting in the Christian tradition and the repetitive, slow, monotone chants of nearly all other religious practices. These chanting practices were included both for their melodious and spiritual significance, as well as the fact that, for most people, the performance of a chant is quite calming and meditative.

Singing can have a very similar effect on the body, allowing you to release stress by working through profound emotional challenges as well as the physical act of modulating and supporting an effective breathing pattern. By all means, sing in the shower, or in the car while stuck in traffic, or right now while reading this book! Music has a very pronounced effect on our autonomic state, and the performance aspect adds the breathing and vocalization components to the effect of music.

Gargling is a unique tool for those who are suffering from digestive issues. When practiced regularly, gargling is very effective in triggering the laryngeal and pharyngeal muscles together as we have the added component of water in our mouth to take into consideration. I recommend that my clients keep a cup by their bathroom sink and include this one-minute exercise in their morning routine when brushing their teeth.

Fill the cup with water (you can optionally add a little bit of salt to the water, as it can help break up mucus at the back of the throat) and take a sip. Hold the water at the back of your throat, and look up and gargle with the water while keeping your mouth open. Gargle for a minimum of 10 seconds per sip of water. Gargle relatively aggressively to fully stimulate the pharyngeal and laryngeal muscles. Your goal should be to gargle hard enough that you begin to have tears coming out of your eyes. This is a sign that the electrical activity in the brain stem is strong enough to activate all four brain stem nuclei involved in VN function.

The physical act of vocalization is quite effective, especially when paired with controlled slower breaths. I recommend implementing one or two of these vocalization practices into your daily routine to help you take advantage of this easily accessible practice in the journey to shift into a parasympathetic state and upgrade your vagus nerve.

THE EFFECT OF MUSIC

Music has a profound effect on us all. The harmonic and melodic frequencies, the beat, the tempo, the bass and treble. There is a scene in the movie *We Are Your Friends*, with actors Zac Efron and Emily Ratajkowski, in which Zac Efron's character, a DJ, is tasked with getting the attendees of a pool party to begin dancing. He explains that the bass line and tempo of the music govern the movement of the body. It's a short scene that is easily found on YouTube to help visualize the effect of music on our bodily functions.

Humans are musical creatures. We have always been attached to music, and it has evolved to help up express our emotions in a deeper way than even words can. Every so often there is a prodigious talent that comes along in the musical sphere and has a profound effect on governing the frequency of our being, just with music. For each of us there are different artists that we connect with at varying levels.

Most of this book was written while I listened to instrumental music paired with a slow, heavy bass line. This is a frequency and beat that helps me get into a productive and creative mindset and is my go-to when I feel the need to use music to help me think or calm down. Some would say that I am able to get lost in this type of music, and I enter a flow state.

There is a lot of individuality when it comes to musical preference (as I continue to learn what my girls prefer to listen to in the car on the way to and from school or at their friends' houses). I encourage you to experiment with how different forms of music and different beats make you feel and find a preferred way to help you calm down to enter that parasympathetic state more effectively. Music affects our breath rate, depth, and quality, which drives autonomic function in either a sympathetic or parasympathetic direction.

NATURE SOUNDS

Nature sounds have been shown to have a calming and relaxing effect on the mind and body. They have been demonstrated to increase HRV through both auditory stimulation and presence in nature, evoking many positive feelings of safety, tranquility, and connectedness. We tend to be able to escape from negative thoughts and distract our cognition effectively when we are outdoors in nature and listen to the sounds of birds chirping, waves crashing, or leaves rustling.

Don't forget that getting outdoors has been shown to have many positive benefits to your health, and the sounds of nature are just a small part of that. We will also discuss the effect of light on our circadian rhythm and, as we well know, sleep is of highest importance in the activation of VN function.

Using individually preferred nature sounds as a relaxation tool and incorporating them into various calm or creative exercises can truly help contribute to parasympathetic activation and overall well-being.

SAFE-AND-SOUND PROTOCOL

The feeling of safety is the most important piece in priming our autonomic state during our development, according to the polyvagal theory proposed by Dr. Stephen Porges. An amazing tool developed by Dr. Porges is a listening therapy protocol called the "Safe and Sound Protocol" (SSP).

According to the polyvagal theory, our autonomic nervous system is constantly searching for clues of safety from our surroundings and the people around us through their body language, facial expression, or tone of voice. Negative past experiences can prime us to have difficulty interpreting these clues effectively, thus causing us to feel threatened more often than we need to.

The SSP utilizes specially filtered music to send cues of safety to your nervous system, shifting your state and allowing you to enter the parasympathetic state of safety more readily. This also allows us to become more social, and as discussed in my previous book, positive social interaction is a great way to build and support VN function.

As you listen to the specially filtered music in the SSP, your nervous system becomes retuned and supports your ability to feel safe and interpret the clues around you correctly. This feeling of safety helps to build resilience and shift your prime state toward parasympathetic.

At the time that I am writing this book, SSP is primarily used in psychology practices to effectively support clients dealing with anxiety, depression, and PTSD, with numerous case studies showing its effective use in children with autism and developmental impairments.

The use of sound therapy is an exciting development due to its ease of application and the amazing case studies that have been published on this therapy. I have begun implementing SSP in my practice and am seeing some very exciting changes in patients feeling more calm and relaxed, and falling asleep more easily. I look forward to seeing more physiological effects in addition to the current applications which are focused on mental health challenges.

CHAPTER 18

TEMPERATURE THERAPY

The regulation of temperature in our living spaces has been a goal for human populations for thousands of years, but artificial tools for regulating that temperature are a relatively recent innovation. Artificial forms of temperature regulation, including indoor heating and cooling devices, especially with the use of electronics, are very effective at monitoring the current temperature and ensuring that our living spaces remain within a specific range. This is certainly a positive from a comfort standpoint; however, it has had some less than ideal effects on our ability to experience and handle variations in temperature.

Constant exposure to temperature-neutral environments, what we today call "room temperature," has caused us to become less resilient to significant variations. I truly believe that the statement "if you don't use it, you'll lose it" is very true when it comes to adaptive physiology and evolutionary biology. The less we expose ourselves to variations, the less resilient we become to handling alterations, thus causing mild changes to become negative stressors. Sitting outside in cooler temperatures and going for walks in more humid environments have become less common, and as such, humans in general have become less adaptive and resilient, particularly in North America.

There is a belief in many parts of the world that being exposed to colder temperatures when one is young, as well as playing and being active in natural environments, will help strengthen the child's immune system. In Nordic countries, it is common practice to have your baby sleep outside for one nap during the day in temperatures as low as -15°C (5°F). Parents report that babies slept longer outside than when in indoor temperatures, and subjective reporting showed that 66 percent of parents found their children to be more active after sleeping outdoors.

It was growing up in this environment that drove Dr. Susanna Søburg, a Danish researcher, to study the use of deliberate exposure to cold or hot environments on our physiology. She is a proponent of using these therapies to help activate mechanisms for health regulation. Her lab's research has opened our eyes to the mechanisms by which temperature changes can have positive effects on our health.

Dr. Søburg's research has found that cold is the most potent stress activator of brown fat, and that any cold exposure that you register as uncomfortable, regardless of the actual temperature, will activate brown fat production. Brown fat has been given this name because it looks brown under a microscope when compared with the more common white fat of adipose tissue. The cause of the brown appearance is due to the presence of higher quantities of mitochondria and iron in these cells, which makes them significantly more metabolically active. The role of brown fat in the body is primarily temperature regulation, as it actively increases metabolism to drive up body temperature. Due to its high metabolic activity, the more brown fat one has, the greater their propensity toward metabolic health. Brown fat is protective against insulin resistance and obesity.

Brown fat is primarily increased through exposure to cold temperatures, as it works to raise body temperature. Deliberate cold exposure is a very effective practice for increasing the quantity of brown fat. Cold air and cold water function differently, as cold air doesn't have quite the rapid effects that cold water does, because we have hairs (even smaller hairs that may not be clearly visible) that create a thin barrier around our bodies, protecting us from cold air. When cold water touches our skin, the hairs are unable to keep their barrier integrity, forcing us to fully experience the cold.

When we either enter a cold plunge or are showered directly with cold water, we rapidly experience a physiological response of sympathetic activation including vasoconstriction (blood vessel narrowing) and signaling to activate the brown fat. The best thing we can do in this circumstance is to focus on our breath. The cold water will immediately feel uncomfortable, and we need to take this opportunity to become comfortable with being uncomfortable. Just as we need to boost our ability to breathe in a slow, nasal, and diaphragmatic manner at rest, this is the next step in the training of our breath—like increasing weights during a workout.[16]

Parasympathetic breathing during deliberate cold exposure is one of the best ways to upgrade your vagus nerve, because you are literally increasing your capacity for high functioning in an uncomfortable environment.

In the opposite direction, deliberate exposure to heat such as sauna therapy is highly beneficial for cardiovascular health and detoxification. Sweating is one of the best ways to release toxins from the body, as sweat is one of three pathways by which toxins are removed (urine and stool being the other two). It also works to trigger vasodilation, the widening of our blood vessels to create resilience in our blood vessels. This has a profound effect on the management of blood pressure, particularly helping to reduce hypertension.[17]

We want to have resilient blood vessels that can effectively switch between vasoconstriction and vasodilation as necessary. As such, the ability to alternate between heat and cold (aka hot-cold cycling) is a great way to build autonomic resilience and detoxify the body, followed by increasing metabolic activity.

Hot-cold cycling is the premise behind many biohacking therapies and thermal spas based in Nordic principles. I've had the opportunity to visit a few spaces and experience hot-cold cycling, and I have to say that this practice has been a big eye-opener and game changer for me. The effects are profound, and regular practice helps to truly build resilience and optimal health.

For best metabolic results, taking a sauna three times per week and splitting up 11 minutes of cold exposure per week (over three or four days) will provide the strongest support for cardiovascular and metabolic health while driving autonomic regulation and parasympathetic activity. Another great study showed an improvement in metabolism with one three-minute cold plunge and five one-minute cold showers per week, so a daily cold plunge is absolutely not a requirement to receive the benefits of cold therapy.[18] Cold showers can be quite effective if taken regularly.

CHAPTER 19

VISUAL THERAPY

How much time do you spend looking at a screen, whether it is your cell phone, computer, television, or tablet? In our more common current lifestyles, we tend to spend a lot of our time staring at our screens with some astounding statistics to prove this.

In 2023, the average American spent 7 hours and 4 minutes looking at their screens each day. Work computers were looked at on average for 2 hours and 51 minutes, and cell phones for 3 hours and 46 minutes. Other screens made up the difference. If we account for 8 hours daily spent sleeping, that increases to over 44 percent of our time looking at screens. Our younger generations are even higher, as Gen Z has been found to be looking at screens for 9 hours each day.[19]

The problem with this is that as we narrow our field of view (the window of focus with our eyes) to look at a screen or to focus on an important point, we actually increase sympathetic activation. Dr. Andrew Huberman has discussed the concept of widening the visual aperture as a technique to activate the parasympathetic nervous system and promote relaxation. He emphasizes the benefits of engaging panoramic vision, which involves taking in a broader field of view to induce a sense of safety and reduce stress.

Dr. Huberman suggests that widening the visual aperture can help shift the nervous system from a state of alertness (associated with the sympathetic nervous system) to a state of relaxation (associated with the parasympathetic nervous system). By intentionally expanding your awareness to include peripheral vision, you can signal to your brain that you are in a safe environment, reducing stress and anxiety. Once again, the concept of feeling safe is utilized to affect physiological changes and shift our state from sympathetic to parasympathetic.

If screen time is inevitable for you because you work on a computer, then the 20-20-20 rule is a great tool to implement to help upgrade VN function. Every 20 minutes, take your eyes off the screen and look at something 20 feet away from you for 20 seconds.[20] This can be paired with standing up or going outside for a break from your screen, but the 20-20-20 rule can help build resilience, improve your feeling of safety, and shift your state to parasympathetic through the day.

Use the 20-20-20 screen time rule to shift your state.

Every 20 minutes, look at an object 20 feet away from you for 20 seconds.

The effect of looking at screens is not simply that it causes you to narrow your visual focus but also that the light produced by screens is what some would call "junk light."

I had Roudy Nassif, the founder of VivaRays on my podcast in early 2022. He explained the concept of protection from junk artificial light, which is a major trigger for stress based on the time that we are looking at screens. When we are outdoors, we are exposed to a full spectrum of light colors. The color of light that we see in the morning at sunrise is very yellow, while the light that we experience in the middle of the day is much more blue and sharp. At sunset, the light color changes to orange and red, which is a prompt for us to want to go to bed.

Screens exude a blue light, especially when backlit by LEDs, which is true for most of our screens these days. Problems tend to occur when we look at our screens first thing in the morning and as we are lying in bed trying to fall asleep. The brightness and color of that light play a profound role in allowing our optimal physiological patterning to occur.

There are three strategies we can utilize to help reduce the effects of junk light from screens each day.

1. Don't look at your screen while you are lying in bed, trying to fall asleep. Try to shut off screen time 60 to 90 minutes before you head to bed. Read a physical book or talk to your significant other during that time instead of sending memes back and forth! Worst case, keep the brightness of your screen as low as possible.

2. Get outside and allow morning sunlight to enter your eyes (don't look directly at the sun, of course!) within 30 minutes of waking up in the morning. This helps to stimulate the production of serotonin in your brain and helps you to feel good and awake during the day.

3. Take breaks from your screens during the day by going outdoors for a walk or to eat your lunch. When we allow sunlight to enter our eyes, it has a profound effect on our physiology and our autonomic state.

I also recommend limiting the use of sunglasses to only when needed, such as driving or in a very bright environment. Sunglasses affect the ability of photons to enter our eyes and create the positive experience of physiological changes.

As discussed, we need to take time away from our screens for multiple reasons, as a narrow gaze and continuous junk light exposure keep us in a sympathetic state and create dysfunction in our physiology.

CHAPTER 20

ADDRESSING CIRCADIAN BIOLOGY

Continuing the discussion on light, we can dive into how to optimize your circadian rhythm.

The circadian rhythm is the natural, internal biological clock that regulates the rhythmic flow of physiological and behavioral processes in a roughly 24-hour cycle. It controls sleep-wake patterns, hormone release, body temperature, and other bodily functions. The circadian rhythm is influenced by external cues like light and darkness, helping to synchronize the body's activities with the day-night cycle.

To optimize this internal clock function, maintaining a consistent sleep schedule and exposure to natural light help keep the circadian rhythm balanced. Light is a key player in the regulation of the circadian rhythm. Brighter light during the day is a direct sign for the body to awaken, while darkness is a direct prompt to us to fall asleep.

What's most important here is to understand that the natural circadian rhythm is involved in allowing us to have strong VN function. The vagus nerve performs many of its recovery functions while we sleep. Most of us are not sleeping nearly enough, which means that we aren't getting VN activity to support recovery during sleep, and this is a by-product of the disruption to our optimal circadian rhythm.

My favorite book on the topic of sleep is *Why We Sleep*, by Matthew Walker. He helps us understand the processes within and necessity of sleep, and why we can no longer take it for granted. We need to optimize our sleep time, and that involves creating habits that allow us to fall asleep easily, stay asleep through the night, and awaken feeling rested and ready to take on the challenge of the next day.

Throughout the night is a great time to assess HRV, as well as first thing in the morning before doing anything that day. While we sleep, VN activity is relatively high, working to support the tissue-resident macrophages in all of our organs and repair any damage of the previous days. As I stated in my previous book, sleep is like the gym for the vagus nerve. Without great quality and adequate timed sleep, the function of VN will be heavily limited during the day and at times when stressors increase.

A couple of wonderful practices that have worked well for some of my clients who had difficulty sleeping are called "yoga nidra" and "non-sleep deep rest" (NSDR) practice. Yoga nidra, also known as "yogic sleep," is a guided meditation technique that induces deep relaxation while maintaining full awareness. It is a systematic practice that allows the subject to enter a state of profound restfulness, akin to the state between wakefulness and sleep.

In a typical yoga nidra session, the person lies down in a comfortable position and follows the instructions of the teacher or recording. The practice involves a series of guided instructions that lead the practitioner through different stages, such as body awareness, breath awareness, and visualization. The goal is to reach a state of deep relaxation, where the body and mind can rest and rejuvenate.

Yoga nidra is used for stress reduction, relaxation, improved sleep, enhanced creativity, and personal growth. Regular practice can help reduce anxiety, promote better sleep, and increase overall well-being.

Non-sleep deep rest (NSDR) involves entering a state of profound restfulness that is distinct from sleep but offers similar benefits. During NSDR, the body and mind experience a state of rest deeper than typical wakefulness, often characterized by reduced brain activity, slowed breathing, and relaxation of muscles.

NSDR practices may include guided meditations, relaxation techniques, and mindfulness exercises designed to induce a state of relaxation and restfulness while maintaining awareness. The goal is to achieve a state of renewal and restoration without the need for a full sleep cycle.

NSDR can be particularly beneficial for individuals who have difficulty falling asleep or those who want to enhance their overall well-being and energy levels. It offers an alternative way to recharge and rejuvenate the body and mind, promoting mental clarity, reduced stress, and improved mood.

Here is a list of the best ways to promote an optimal circadian rhythm:

- Stop eating food at least two hours before going to sleep.
- Stop using your phone for at least one hour before bedtime.
- Use blue-light-blocking apps or glasses if you can't get off your phone until late.
- Keep the lights in your home dim after the sun sets in the evening.

- Get your eyes in natural sunlight within 30 minutes of waking up.
- Sleep in a cool and very dark room.
- Spend time outdoors during daylight to provide your eyes with natural sunlight at different times throughout the day.
- Stick to a similar bedtime and wake-up time daily, including weekdays and weekends.
- Practice five minutes of slow, nasal breathing as you fall asleep.

Start by determining which current habits are stopping you from getting great sleep. Focus on making one or two changes to the lowest hanging fruit, because this will likely have a profound effect on your ability to fall asleep easily and get great rest every night, while upgrading your vagus nerve.

CASE STUDY: MARY

Mary is one of my most inspiring clients. She is a 62-year-old mother of four young men. When she first came to see me, she shared her story and had me in tears. When she was just a child, her father kidnapped her and multiple other girls and held them captive for many years. There was significant abuse and trauma inflicted upon her during this time, and her father's case became one of the most infamous kidnapping cases in Canada in the 1970s. She had surgical reconstruction to repair trauma to her face and suffered significant emotional challenges for years following. Mary then was involved in a catastrophic car accident at age 42 in which she lost a significant amount of brain function and had a significant reduction in her vision, causing her to become legally blind.

What is inspiring about her case was her resolve. She became interested in the vagus nerve and immediately reached out to me for support in helping her overcome her mounting health challenges. Low energy, excess body weight, cognitive fog challenges, sleep apnea, and the beginning stages of liver cirrhosis were all diagnosed in the past decade. She had even suffered giardiasis from a parasite 15 years prior to seeing me.

We immediately began to look into her current cellular and gastrointestinal function to determine if there were biochemical challenges that we could address. We also brought her into our online group coaching program to support her social connectedness, something that had been very challenging for her during the COVID lockdowns—she had not seen her four sons in nearly three years.

We helped her address some nutritional deficiencies but focused on stress management and VN activation exercises such as breathing and optimizing her circadian biology. She began walking outside daily for 1.5 to 2 hours in the morning sunlight—a challenging feat considering she lived in a northern climate that has snow approximately seven months of the year.

Mary began to notice improvement in her health quite quickly, with fluctuations on a daily basis, but she was excited to see some positive changes that she kept at the forefront of her mind. She was also able to create some boundaries in her family life that were holding her back from achieving happiness in her home environment. Soon after, she was able to start seeing her children again!

I've been working with Mary for one year, and the changes are exciting to see. She has reduced her body weight from 175 lbs. to 138 lbs. Her mental clarity and cognition is significantly improved overall, and she has much less chronic pain, such that she was able to reduce CBD dosage by 60 percent, which she'd used for sleep and pain management. Mary has even decreased the use of her white cane when going to the grocery store or around the neighborhood.

She attributes much of her success to her daily time outside in the morning sunlight, a practice that has helped to recalibrate her circadian rhythm, her hormones, and her metabolism. Most importantly, she is happy. Mary shares with our group participants on a weekly basis that even though she feels like a tornado is happening around her, she is so much happier and more confident due to her new outlook on life!

CHAPTER 21

CREATIVE PURSUITS

I was in a Lego store with my daughter and her friend some months ago when a middle-aged gentleman walked by me holding three boxes that he was purchasing. One was a Star Wars Death Star, the second was the Batmobile, and the last was Captain America's shield from the Avengers. He caught me looking at the boxes, turned to me, and said, "Lego calms the mind."

I was a bit stunned when this happened, as I didn't think much of it other than I hadn't realized Lego was partnered with so many different brands, but his comment caught me off guard. It also prompted me to consider the concept of creative pursuits and their effects on our physiology.

Creative pursuits can involve anything from interpretive dance to adult coloring books, puzzles, writing, and yes, even building 1,500-piece Lego sets. As with so many other concepts, there is a lot of individuality in what one would choose to pursue, not to say that you are limited to just one creative pursuit at any time.

While we are in a creative flow state, our physiology knows that we are safe. We can only truly enter a flow state of creativity when we feel safe, and so this is a wonderful practice to implement in whatever way you personally see fit. Your creative pursuit doesn't have to even have an outcome attached to it, other than allowing you to spend time sharing your unique gifts with yourself or the world.

At Health Upgraded, our goal is to help you achieve optimal health so that your health challenges no longer hold you back from sharing your unique gifts with the world. We believe that human ingenuity is the driving force of our success, and so we want to help remove or lower the barrier of poor health that may be holding you back. Creative pursuits are highly linked to this process, so engaging in these practices can be such a breath of fresh air for your body, especially if you tend to be in a sympathetic, hypersensitive state. Take some time to reengage your creativity and connect with your inner child. We are all allowed to play, no matter our age!

CONCLUSION

It has been a pleasure to demystify the amazing vagus nerve for you. Throughout this book, we delved into the intricate connection between your vagus nerve and the various aspects of your physical, emotional, and mental health. You have learned that the vagus nerve is not merely a messenger that carries signals between your brain and body, but it's a conductor of harmony that orchestrates the symphony of your internal systems. By tending to your vagus nerve, you have the remarkable ability to influence your digestion, immunity, heart rate, stress response, and even your emotional resilience.

It is essential to remember that the journey you've undertaken is not about seeking quick fixes or external solutions. Rather, it is about cultivating a deep understanding of your own body and mind and embracing the wisdom of holistic well-being. The practices and techniques shared in this book are not intended to be fleeting interventions but rather integral components of a sustainable lifestyle that nurtures your ability to rebound from all forms of stress.

As you've explored the practices of breathwork, meditation, mindful movement, and social engagement, you've become attuned to the subtleties of your body's responses. You've recognized that every breath you take, every moment of presence you cultivate, and every connection you foster has the potential to enhance the vitality of your vagus nerve. Through your journey, you've experienced the power of the mind-body connection and witnessed firsthand how your thoughts and emotions can shape your physiological state.

However, embracing change and transformation is not always easy. It requires dedication, patience, and a willingness to face the discomfort that might arise when stepping out of familiar patterns. Remember that growth is a continuous process, and setbacks are an integral part of the journey. When faced with challenges, approach them with the same compassion and curiosity that you've extended to yourself throughout this exploration. Your vagus nerve thrives on your ability to adapt and evolve, and every step you take toward embracing change contributes to its vitality.

I encourage you to view this book not as the end of your journey but as a new beginning. Integrate the exercises and practices into your daily routines, weave them into the fabric of your relationships, and let them guide you toward upgraded health.

As you move forward, remain open to the signals your body sends you. Listen to the whispers of your vagus nerve—those gentle nudges and intuitive sensations that guide you toward choices that align with your well-being. Just as a skilled sailor learns to read the wind and tides, you too can become attuned to the rhythms of your own body, navigating the currents of life with grace and intention.

It is my sincere hope that *Upgrade Your Vagus Nerve* has served as a road map for your journey toward optimal health and vitality. I am honored to have been your guide as you explored the vast landscape of your inner world. Remember that your vagus nerve is not merely an anatomical structure but a metaphorical bridge that connects your inner and outer worlds. By tending to this bridge, you harmonize the two, allowing the energy of wellness to flow freely.

The potential lies within you, waiting to be activated. Embrace the practices, insights, and wisdom you've gained on your journey to vitality, resilience, and profound well-being.

With gratitude,

Dr. Navaz Habib

For an up-to-date list of Dr. Habib's favorite resources to *Upgrade the Vagus Nerve*, please visit www.healthupgraded.com/resources.

ENDNOTES

1 Stephen Porges, *The Polyvagal Theory: Neurophysiological Foundations of Emotions, Attachment, Communication, and Self-Regulation*, New York: W. W. Norton & Co., 2011.

2 M. Canyelles, C. Borràs, N. Rotllan, M. Tondo, J. C. Escolà-Gil, and F. Blanco-Vaca, "Gut Microbiota-Derived TMAO: A Causal Factor Promoting Atherosclerotic Cardiovascular Disease?," *International Journal of Molecular Sciences* 24, no. 3 (January 18, 2023), https://doi.org/10.3390/ijms24031940.

3 K. A. Böckmann, A. R. Franz, M. Minarski, et al., "Differential Metabolism of Choline Supplements in Adult Volunteers," *European Journal of Nutrition* 61 (July 21, 2021): 219–230, https://doi.org/10.1007/s00394-021-02637-6.

4 X. Ma, et al., "Excessive Intake of Sugar: An Accomplice of Inflammation," *Frontiers in Immunology* 13 (August 2022).

5 F. Jameel, M. Phang, L. G. Wood, and M. L. Garg, "Acute Effects of Feeding Fructose, Glucose, and Sucrose on Blood Lipid Levels and Systemic Inflammation," *Lipids in Health and Disease* 13 (December 16, 2014): 195, https://www.ncbi.nlm.nih.gov/pmc/articles/PMC4290803.

6 C. S. Dweck, *Mindset*, Chicago: Ballantine Books, 2008.

7 B. A. Bari et al., "Locus Coeruleus-Norepinephrine: Basic Functions and Insights into Parkinson's Disease," *Neural Regeneration Research* 15, no. 6 (June 2020): 1006–13, doi: 10.4103/1673-5374.270297.

8 B. N. Keller, A. E. Snyder, C. R. Coker, E. A. Aguilar, M. K. O'Brien, S. S. Bingaman, A. C. Arnold, A. Hajnal, and Y. Silberman, "The Vagus Nerve Is Critical for Regulation of Hypothalamic-Pituitary-Adrenal Axis Responses to Acute Stress," Preprint, 2021, https://www.biorxiv.org/content/10.1101/2021.06.03.446790v1.

9 U. Moens et. al, "The c-fos cAMP-Response Element: Regulation of Gene Expression by a Beta 2-adrenergic Agonist, Serum, and DNA Methylation," *Biochimica et biophysica acta* (1993): 63–70.

10 M. Skok, "Mitochondrial Nicotinic Acetylcholine Receptors: Mechanisms of Functioning and Biological Significance," *The International Journal of Biochemistry & Cell Biology* (2022): 143.

11 "Hippocrates Quotes," Goodreads, accessed October 2023, https://www.goodreads.com/author/quotes/248774.

12 C. R. Cole, E. H. Blackstone, F. J. Pashkow, C. E. Snader, and M. S. Lauer, "Heart-Rate Recovery Immediately after Exercise as a Predictor of Mortality," *New England Journal of Medicine* 341, no. 18 (October 19, 1999): 1351–7.

13 Partrick McKeown, *The Oxygen Advantage*.

14 electroCore Inc. "Study Presented at 75th Annual Meeting of the American Academy of Neurology Demonstrates that gammaCore (nVNS) Can Accelerate Foreign Language Learning," April 24, 2023, accessed August 22, 2023, https://www.globenewswire.com/en/news-release/2023/04/24 /2652647/0/en/Study-Presented-at-75th-Annual-Meeting-of-the -American-Academy-of-Neurology-Demonstrates-that-gammaCore -nVNS-Can-Accelerate-Foreign-Language-Learning.html.

15 L. K. McIntire, R. A. McKinley, C. Goodyear, J. P. McIntire, and R. D. Brown, "Cervical Transcutaneous Vagal Nerve Stimulation (ctVNS) Improves Human Cognitive Performance under Sleep Deprivation Stress," *Communications Biology* 4, no. 1 (June 10, 2021): 634, https://doi.org/10.1038 /s42003-021-02145-7.

16 S. Søberg, J. Löfgren, F. E. Philipsen, M. Jensen, A. E. Hansen, E. Ahrens, K. B. Nystrup, et al., "Altered Brown Fat Thermoregulation and Enhanced Cold-Induced Thermogenesis in Young, Healthy, Winter-Swimming Men," *Cell Reports Medicine* 2, no. 10 (October 11, 2021): 100408. doi: 10.1016/j.xcrm .2021.100408.

17 K. N. Henderson, L. G. Killen, E. K. O'Neal, and H. S. Waldman, "The Cardiometabolic Health Benefits of Sauna Exposure in Individuals with High-Stress Occupations. A Mechanistic Review," *International Journal of Environmental Research and Public Health* 18, no. 3 (January 27, 2021): 1105, https://www.mdpi.com/1660-4601/18/3/1105.

18 P. Šrámek, M. Šimečková, L. Janský, J. Savlíková, and S. Vybíral, "Human Physiological Responses to Immersion into Water of Different Temperatures," *European Journal of Applied Physiology* 81, no. 5 (March 2000): 436–42. doi: 10.1007/s004210050065.

19 S. Zauderer, *Average Screen Time Statistics & Facts*, accessed August 12, 2023, https://www.crossrivertherapy.com/research/screen-time -statistics#:~:text=The%20average%20American%20spends%20 7,favorite%20TV%20shows%20and%20movies.

20 B. Chou, "Deconstructing the 20-20-20 Rule for Digital Eye Strain," *Optom Times* (2018): 21–23.

GRATITUDE

First and foremost, my wife Noureen, my daughters Miraal and Misha—I love you all so much. Thank you for always being my first-line supporters and my reason!

Next, my parents and in-laws—thank you for all you do to support our family; you guys are the best!

The Health Upgraded team—Saima, Laura, Emma—you are all so wonderful and powerful. Your support means the world, and I know I couldn't do all that I do without you all.

To all my mentors and supporters along the way, thank you for your guidance, and for the push to be better and to do better.

Lastly, to JP, Gary, Mitch, and the team at electroCore—you guys rock! Thank you for reigniting my passion and handing me the reins to share our messages in conjunction!

Love and gratitude to you all.

ABOUT THE AUTHOR

Dr. Navaz Habib is the founder of Health Upgraded, a functional medicine and health optimization clinic in Toronto, Canada, working with high-performing professionals, athletes, and entrepreneurs to dig a little deeper and find the answers to what is holding back their health. He works with those who want to take their health to a higher level, allowing them to contribute to humanity and serve more people.

Having gone through his own personal experiences with poor health and weight struggles, Dr. Habib is well equipped to implement personalized recommendations for each of his clients. In identifying the root causes of health imbalances and addressing them naturally, his patients experience optimal health the way their bodies were meant to feel; this allows them to give back to the world in whatever way they want to serve.

By activating the vagus nerve, you can optimize your productivity, focus, and energy levels, allowing you to experience the effects of upgraded health.

To learn more about his work, visit his websites www.healthupgraded .com or www.drnavazhabib.com and connect with him on Instagram @DrNavazHabib.

Printed in the USA
CPSIA information can be obtained
at www.ICGtesting.com
CBHW060025140624
9935CB00008B/30

9 781646 046188